Reiki Healing for Beginners

Self Help Guide to Increase Energy and Heal Your Mind and Body With Reiki Healing

(Cure Yourself With From Anxiety, Insomnia, Depression, Chronic Pain and Panic Attacks)

Rose Brennan

Published by Rob Miles

Rose Brennan

All Rights Reserved

Reiki Healing for Beginners: Self Help Guide to Increase Energy and Heal Your Mind and Body With Reiki Healing (Cure Yourself With From Anxiety, Insomnia, Depression, Chronic Pain and Panic Attacks)

ISBN 978-1-989990-52-0

All rights reserved. No part of this guide may be reproduced in any form without permission in writing from the publisher except in the case of brief quotations embodied in critical articles or reviews.

Legal & Disclaimer

The information contained in this book is not designed to replace or take the place of any form of medicine or professional medical advice. The information in this book has been provided for educational and entertainment purposes only.

The information contained in this book has been compiled from sources deemed reliable, and it is accurate to the best of the Author's knowledge; however, the Author cannot guarantee its accuracy and validity and cannot be held liable for any errors or omissions. Changes are periodically made to this book. You must consult your doctor or get professional medical advice before using any of the suggested remedies, techniques, or information in this book.

Upon using the information contained in this book, you agree to hold harmless the Author from and against any damages, costs, and expenses, including any legal fees potentially resulting from the application of any of the information provided by this guide. This disclaimer applies to any damages or injury caused by the use and application, whether directly or indirectly, of any advice or information presented, whether for breach of contract, tort, negligence, personal injury, criminal intent, or under any other cause of action.

You agree to accept all risks of using the information presented inside this book. You need to consult a professional medical practitioner in order to ensure you are both able and healthy enough to participate in this program.

Table of Contents

INTRODUCTION 1

CHAPTER 1: WHAT IS REIKI? 5

CHAPTER 2: REIKI ATTUNEMENT 9

CHAPTER 3: WHAT IS ENERGY - EXISTENCE THEORY 19

CHAPTER 4: BASIC BIOENERGETICS 30

CHAPTER 5: RESEARCH AND GENERAL ACKNOWLEDGEMENT 40

CHAPTER 6: WHAT IS REIKI? 56

CHAPTER 7: REIKI'S NEGATIVE SIDE 60

CHAPTER 8: IS REIKI VITALITY RECUPERATING CRAFTSMANSHIP A TRUE BLUE PRACTICE? 63

CHAPTER 9: THE SACRAL CHAKRA 73

CHAPTER 10: ADDITIONAL REIKI PROTECTION AND CLEANSING 78

CHAPTER 11: CREATING THE ATMOSPHERE FOR WORKSHOPS/ATTUNING 95

CHAPTER 12: THE HISTORY OF REIKI 105

CHAPTER 13: REIKI TREATMENT METHOD - THE MOST POWERFUL SPIRITUAL HEALING ARTS YET VERY SMOOTH AND HEALTHY 130

CHAPTER 14: THE FIFTH CHAKRA 140

CHAPTER 15: YOGA FOR HEALTH PROBLEMS 144

CHAPTER 16: WHAT IS ILLNESS? 151

CHAPTER 17: CHAKRAS.. 163

CHAPTER 18: REIKI PRACTICE AND GROWTH OF INTUITIVE ABILITIES 192

CONCLUSION.. 200

Introduction

You may not be aware of it, but yoga is more than a system of exercise. In fact, I would go as far as saying that it is a way of life. If you have found that your life is unsatisfactory and want to feel some inner joy, then yoga may be exactly what the doctor ordered. More and more people are turning to natural ways to stem their negativity and to find inner peace because it's a healthier way of dealing with the lack in lifestyle than turning to traditional medicines. In fact, traditional medicines are failing. When you see how many US residents are being prescribed anti-depressant drugs and try to put that together with the increase in depression related illnesses, it doesn't make sense that people are choosing a method which has proven to be ineffective. Yoga, however, has been proven to give inner peace and has been used for centuries.

The thing that may be putting you off yoga is the fact that you believe it is related to religion or that there are only certain types of people who do it. You may see it as some trendy kind of fad and dismiss the importance of it, but if you have any sense at all, you have to admit that those practicing it are doing so because it improves their lives. Look on YouTube and other places and you will find that the benefits of yoga are so all encompassing that they cover mental health, physical wellbeing and mobility and can help with all of these. This book takes the mystery out of it and explains to the layman what yoga is all about, how it can help you to gain inner peace, how you can meditate and what it is doing to your body.

Take the course of your life into your own hands and you begin to see that you have a lot more power than you may have thought. That power lies in the way that you sit, the way that you breathe – but most of all in the way that you think. The book will take you through a little bit about yoga and where it comes from, but it won't dwell too much on that. It is intended to guide you and to help you to incorporate yoga into your life because when you do, you will find your life improves dramatically. You become more tolerant, you feel better in yourself, you breathe in a more conscious way and your body responds by feeling well. The inner peace that you achieve is as a direct result of your efforts.

As we walk you through the stages that will help you to incorporate yoga into your life, you need to understand that yoga is not an exercise routine. It isn't something that you have to hurry or that has to hurt you in order to do you any good. Instead, it's a change of lifestyle. You live yoga, you don't just do it. When you do, you find that your mind is more open to all the possibilities that life holds out to you, that you may not otherwise have noticed. Your life will become richer and your understanding of life more enlightened.

Chapter 1: What Is Reiki?

Reiki healing is an ancient practice that has been carried out for more than a thousand years. Many adherents believe Reiki healing was first practiced by Tibetan Buddhist monks and was only revived by Dr. Mikao Usui, a Japanese Buddhist, during the late part of the 19*th* century. Dr. Usui then developed his own Reiki system, also referred to as Usui system, which is an incredibly simple, yet potent method of healing. Reiki can be effortlessly bestowed and received by any person who is willing to learn the practice.

The term Reiki was derived from **Rei**, which means universal and **Ki**. which means life force or energy. **Ki** is believed to be the energy that everything here on earth is made of. It can be likened to **Chi,** which the Chinese believe in. **Ki** is the primary energy that is present in all things, whether they exist in the physical plane or in the other planes of consciousness.

Reiki is an extraordinary type of healing energy that can only be controlled by a person who has reached attunement with it. The process of attuning or initiating a person to Reiki healing is the continuation of a very old practice of aligning a person with the healing energies of Reiki by utilizing the holy Reiki symbols that were made known to Mikao Usui. When a person has been attuned, he or she becomes a channel for Reiki healing energy for the rest of his or her life. A newly attuned healer will feel an unusual surge of energy within him or her.

Reiki energy is a healing energy that stirs within the healer's being, which is then spiritually transferred to the person requiring some form of healing. Even though Reiki energy is transferred to the recipient, the healer does not really diminish his own level of Reiki energy. As a matter of fact, the more a healer heals other people, the more he is energized and becomes healed himself. Reiki energy is deemed as an "intelligent energy" because it goes to the exact location where its healing power is needed through the spiritual guidance of the healer.

All forms of healing people do employs a universal energy to treat a person with illness. But Reiki healing is different because it is only used for the achievement of the greater good. You can never really abuse or misuse Reiki energy. An attuned healer will be able to perform Reiki treatments simply by having the intention to heal and placing his or her hands on the person who requires a certain form of healing. Although there are specific hand positions that the Reiki healer needs to learn to administer the process, the Reiki energy is able to naturally flow to the exact location where healing is required and the healer does not have to consciously direct the energy to flow.

Chapter 2: Reiki Attunement

Receiving a Reiki attunement is the one prerequisite for practicing Reiki and for channeling Reiki energy. The ability to channel Reiki - to have Reiki healing energy flow into you and through you - is passed on from Reiki Master to student. As mentioned previously, Dr. Usui was the first person to develop a method for adjusting a person's energy pathways to accommodate the flow of Reiki. He passed the ability to attune down to his students – the original Reiki Masters. Only a Reiki Master can conduct an attunement.

The ability to channel Reiki is already within you, and within every human being. The Reiki Master's role during attunement is drawing back the curtains, or opening a door, thus letting the energy flow into a space that already existed within you.

The attunement process can be very profound. It may be felt as a powerful spiritual experience or it can feel subtler. The experience during the attunement is not as important. What is important is that you now have the ability to channel Reiki energy and the ability to heal yourself and others with Reiki.

During the attunement the Reiki Master is guided by the universal energy to open the student's energy channels or spiritual chakras to Reiki energy, and then joins the student to this energy flow. Once joined to the Reiki source, you, the student, will be attuned to Reiki and have the ability to use Reiki for the rest of your life. You can never lose Reiki. Even without any further training, you can begin to heal with Reiki. Remember, Reiki cannot do harm. It has its own universal intelligence and is self-directed in healing. You merely need to place your hands with an intent to heal through Reiki. With that intention in place,

Reiki will begin to flow through you and know exactly where to go and what to do. Reiki can and will move through the chakras/aura to heal, however, it does not always move beyond your hand location. This is why it can be important for beginners to use all the hand positions (described later in this book) before using a more intuitive approach.

The best advice while giving Reiki is to relax, give a healing intent, and know that Reiki is guided by the universal consciousness and will do all it needs – never causing harm, only bringing healing, safety and love. You can remove yourself from the process and know that by acting with healing intent to channel Reiki, you have done all you need to do. Reiki will do the rest.

Likewise, when receiving Reiki, you can merely be open to receiving the healing energy and know that in the wisdom of universal ki, you will be given all you need for vibrant health and wellness.

Reiki Levels

Reiki Level 1

The first Reiki level. Students receive one, two, or four attunements, learn the history of Reiki, learn the Reiki hand positions, and practice self-treatment and treatment of others. Class takes 1-2 days.

Reiki Level 2

The second Reiki level. Students receive two attunements. Students learn how to give distant treatments. The first three Reiki symbols are revealed and taught. Class takes 2 days.

Reiki Level 3

The third Reiki level. Students receive one attunement- the Master level attunement.

Students learn the master and completion symbols. Students meet for five weeks.

The image shows the flow of Reiki after each level/attunement.

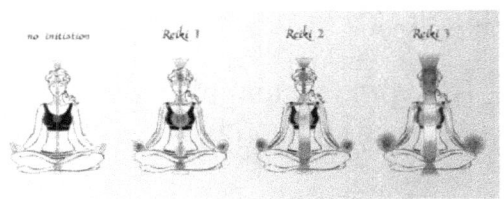

Choosing A Reiki Master For Your Attunement/Classes

A Reiki Master (or sensei/teacher) is a Reiki practitioner who has reached the highest level of practice and empowerment and is able to attune students to Reiki. They have gone through Reiki Level 1, Level 2, Level 3, and have received the Master level attunement, been shown the Master symbol, and been taught how to pass on the attunement. A

Reiki Master must be able to show his/her direct lineage of attunement down from Master Usui. Do not go to a Level 1 workshop if the Reiki Master cannot show their attunement lineage. Below are a few questions to consider when choosing a Reiki Master.

What is your lineage? What other credentials do you have?

How long have you been practicing Reiki?

How long is the workshop?

What is covered in the workshop? Topics? Materials?

How many attunements do you give your students?

How much hands-on practice will we have during the workshop?

How much do you charge?

Are you part of any professional organizations?

What levels of Reiki do you teach? I, II, III?

Do you provide professional Reiki treatments?

Do I receive a certificate of completion?

How many students are typically in the workshop?

Are you available for questions/concerns/etc. after the class is over?

After interviewing your potential teacher, you may feel ready to sign up for the class. You may also consider receiving a Reiki treatment from the teacher before signing up. Importantly, you must feel comfortable with the teacher and their teaching style.

The Reiki Symbols

The Reiki Symbols are a powerful tool in Reiki healing. However, the symbols are not necessary to give Reiki healing (there are no symbols in the first degree).

The Reiki symbols are only given to students who have taken and been attuned to Reiki Level II. They are sacred and are meant to be kept confidential. There are images of the symbols available on the internet, however, before the internet the symbols were kept secret by burning the pages they were drawn on at the end of each class. Although they are available for anyone to see, the power of the symbol only works after a student has been attuned or opened to it in the Reiki Level II attunement.

The symbols are as follows:

Cho Ku Rei

The Power Symbol, known as Cho Ku Rei, amplifies or gives more power to the Reiki treatment or any thought, action, or outcome. It has many uses, but the intended purpose is to empower, or frequently, strengthen Reiki healing.

Sei Hei Ki

The Harmony or Emotional/Mental Symbol is used to help anyone dealing with emotional pain, relationship troubles, mental health difficulties, addiction, or bad habits.

Hon Sha Ze Sho Nen

The Connection or Distant Healing Symbol extends to allow Reiki Practitioners conduct healings in absentia. They can channel Reiki to others across town, across the country, or across an ocean. This symbol connects the practitioner to the receiver.

These three symbols are taught in Reiki Level II.

Key Take Away

To practice Reiki, you must be attuned or empowered by a Reiki Master. This typically occurs in a Level 1 Reiki Class. Once you have been opened to the flow of Reiki you are ready to start healing with Reiki. You do not need to know what to do – merely allow the Reiki to guide you and Reiki will do the rest.

There are three levels of Reiki. Reiki symbols, which increase the potency of Reiki, are taught in Level II.

Chapter 3: What Is Energy - Existence Theory

When studying Reiki, understanding our existence in the broadest sense of the word does not require that we answer existential questions like where we came from, how we got here and where we are going. We need only consider our existence in one single moment. Now.

In the "Now" we exist as something that our science has already been able to determine with undeniable certainty.

Energy.

Everything in the universe that exists, no matter its shape, is that.

Science has also determined that Energy is never ending and have always existed. This is based on the certainty that Energy can be changed, but cannot be created or destroyed. This means that the universal "quantity" of energy that exists now, has and always will be the same. Only it's form (pattern) changes.

Considering our existence on a micro level, it is clear that we exist because we have a certain pattern of energy. A structural pattern that results in an identifiable entity.

This pattern and it's inherent connectivity is so potent that it combines into a living breathing physical being. One with skin and bones and organs. One with memories and cognitive abilities. A being that has the ability to affect the world around it.

It is also clear that it does not exist in isolation. It lives in a world that it can affect, and that affects it's existence often in unexpected ways.

Balance

When we consider energy in it's most basic form, it exists in one or a combination of two states. In balance or out of balance.

The simplest way to understand what this means is to understand what imbalance means.

Imbalance for this purpose means "causing motion". Whenever there is motion, it is caused by imbalance. When there is no motion, there is a state of balance or equilibrium.

E.g. Rivers flow because water wants to move to the lowest point. At the top, the water is in a state of imbalance. Water flowing downwards is a corrective action. When it reaches the lowest point, it will form a lake. The river is water out of balance attempting to correct its own state of imbalance. The lake is water, in a state of balance, after completion of the corrective action (motion toward balance).

When we look at the universe on a macro scale it is clear that there is always an imbalance somewhere.

No matter what the cause is or where the imbalance exists, there is also always a corrective action. Movement or change occurs with the sole purpose of correcting imbalance. The knock-on affect will result in a change causing a new imbalance somewhere else. This cycle of imbalance to balance and back is never-ending.

Conversely, if there were no imbalances anywhere, nothing would ever happen. The universe would be in a complete state of equilibrium and therefore completely static.

As a Reiki practitioner you are manipulating the balance of the energy in the environment that you are working in. Your energy work will either focus on creating or correcting an imbalance.

The Connection of Everything

The only way imbalance can continuously exist is if all the change causing affects are connected together. The river would have nowhere to flow if not for the sloped river bed containing it.

Everything is connected to everything and nothing lives in isolation. This means that if you threw a small stone in the ocean a thousand miles away the ripples in the water are connected to you. The affect of those ripples on you from a thousand miles away would likely not be significant, however, by virtue of the connection of everything between you and the stone, you will be affected in some way.

No matter how big or small an imbalance, it is connected to everything and will have an affect on everything.

The Mass of Everything

The more energy something has, the more mass it contains. The more mass it contains the more it's ability to affect the world around it.

E.g. When you throw a rubber ball at a window, chances are it will just bounce back. When you throw a ball made of steel the same size, the window will likely be broken.

No matter the significance of the energy, it has mass. Even thoughts have mass. Generally not significant but since energy is everything and thoughts do exist, they do have mass.

Some thoughts have more mass than others. Thoughts directly connected with strong emotions, tend to be "bigger", containing more energy and therefore more mass. Think about the last time you were really angry, or really happy.

When you think of a thought as a pebble being dropped in the universal energy ocean, the bigger the pebble, the bigger the ripples.

This is an important lesson to learn. Skill at empowering your healing practice with the right mass, will dramatically increase your abilities.

Life

As a Reiki practitioner you will be dealing with living (animate) things. People, animals and even plants. In the context of existence theory, life is defined as "Energy in continuous motion". When motion stops due to an established state of balance, life ceases and the body becomes inanimate (dead).

Life does not require an additional external force to create imbalance to sustain motion. Life is the imbalance.

Life does not exist in isolation however. In order to sustain it's imbalance It is connected to the world around it. It needs physical things to survive like oxygen, food and water. Even when those things are withheld, life will continue for at least for a little while.

Because life is energy continuously in motion, it is ever changing, growing, developing and never stationary. The beauty of it's existence and the sheer power of it's continuation driven by what makes so.

When the body of a living creature dies (becomes inanimate), the energy patterns that were responsible for animation of that body, does not cease to exist. That would be impossible. It continues to exists as something that is identifiable as that creature. This is generally referred to as the spirit.

What makes it identifiable as you are your memories which are uniquely combined in a way that can only be you.

Combining body and spirit, the body provides the spirit with some very important physical abilities. These are purely biologically and electro-chemically driven abilities and are used to connect and interact with the world around you.

When we consider the body and spirit separately, we find that the ability to think, reason and experience emotions are those bio- and electro-chemically driven features of physical body.

Trying to account for the element that make you identifiable as you, your memories, is a little more complicated. Studies have attempted to identify the physical location of memories in the brain and have failed. Memories that were thought to be located in specific centers in the brain were recuperated even when those parts of the brain were damaged and rendered unusable. This means that the memories reside outside of the physical body. The spirit.

This also means that memories are static. Once made they do not change. There may be circumstances where memories are perceived to have changed. These perceptions are incorrect. An existing memory may be overlaid with a new one, however, the overlaid memory now becomes a new memory. The old memory continues to exist as well.

Since an inanimate body and a static spirit are both in a state of equilibrium, for life to exist there needs to be an interaction between the energetic body (with it's physical abilities) and the spirit body (your memories). This interaction is what causes the imbalance that sparks life.

Without the presence of a body, a spirit and an interaction between the two, animated life as we know it does not exist.

Chapter 4: Basic Bioenergetics

Reiki is included in what is being called energy therapies. I prefer to use the word "bioenergetic" because I consider that in many cases these therapies handle terms that are difficult to identify with what is commonly understood by energy (electric, magnetic, light, heat, etc.). Within the concept of "bioenergy", we will understand "non-material influences" of different types that exert their effects on humans in very different ways. These influences in the West have been called energy. Probably trying to make use of the concept of "energy" as opposed to that of "matter". In this way, all those who do not use a material vehicle directly to exert their effect are considered as energy therapies. In other cases, the concept of the "spiritual" is used as opposed to the "material". Thus, it is common to mix or not differentiate energy and spiritual therapies. In this manual, we will use the term "bioenergetic" to refer to both one and the other and we will see that Reiki can fit into both classifications.

The "non-material influences" I referred to have been contemplated by different cultures since ancient times. Some of these influences have been understood and explained, more or less completely, by science. Some examples may be solar radiation or natural radiation of different types, which influence the state of health in different ways. In other cases, these influences turned out to be "non-tangible" rather than "non-material". The clearest example may be that of microorganisms or germs present in certain diseases. Science has studied many of these "energies" by giving them names and explaining them to a greater or lesser extent, but there are others, of which ancient cultures speak to us, but to which science has not given a definitive explanation or cataloging.

Each culture has given these influences different names and has given them an explanation from their cosmology. In this sense it is interesting to note that in the West there has been a separation between cosmology (study of the physical universe) and metaphysics (study of the spirit), but in other cultures the spirit is inherent in the physical world, so that the one does not It can be understood without the other.

Today many people are interested in studying the knowledge that comes to us from these ancient cultures, assimilating or understanding them from our own mentality, thus creating "Western bioenergetics".

This knowledge comes to us impregnated in the language and spirituality of these countries, and their understanding and adaptation to our way of life, our religious concept, and our science are complicated on many occasions.

In the effort to access the information contained in this knowledge it happens that sometimes we distort and confuse their meaning. Other times we find that the approaches made to us from these traditions seem to directly contradict what our science and culture teaches us, making reconciliation impossible. In other cases, more than it may seem, we can observe how the human being has understood since ancient times things that only recently science dares to raise, being the old permits perfectly identifiable with current scientific approaches.

If we ignore possible frauds, purely personal opinions, and intentionally falsified information, all the Cosmo-logical approaches that we find in other ancient cultures are compatible, in one way or another, with current scientific knowledge. It is only necessary to be able to see the pyramid from all angles and understand that there is the last vertex that unites all the ways of seeing the Universe: the need to understand the outer and inner world, the ultimate reality and thus be able to approach the state of balance longed for by the human being.

Of the cosmological systems that come to us from other cultures, some of them attract attention because of their apparent globality, universality and practical immediacy. Among them, we can highlight two that have been mostly chosen: the Tantric and Taoist culture. The one and the others have reached the West by the hand of Yoga and Traditional Chinese Medicine, two practices that we have adopted in our culture as an alternative means of enhancing our health.

Orginally the ultimate goal of one and another system is not limited to seeking the improvement of the health of the individual. What we find in his teachings and practices is a description of the manifestation of the spirit in this world and tools to achieve its total integration into our lives. For what purpose? Reach the state of harmony in each and every aspect of our life and come to live with a special connection with the universe. This total harmony will be, from now on, what we will consider as integral health.

Probably, of these two knowledge sectors, the closest to Reiki is Taoist. Its founder, the Japanese Mikao Usui, was a student of esoteric Buddhism arrived in Japan from China. One of the disciplines he studied during his youth was the Kiko, a variant of the Chinese Qi Gong. The Qi Gong is one of the disciplines encompassed in Traditional Chinese Medicine, deeply influenced by the Taoist view of nature. One of the practices of Kiko is the accumulation of Ki (a concept that we will discuss later) in the body in order to use it to strengthen one's health or transmit it to other people for healing. Possibly in this practice is the root of what would later be the Usui Reiki Ryoho. Studying the Taoist conception of nature and health, we are probably studying the basis on which Usui supported his natural healing system, so this will be one of the driving pillars of this manual.

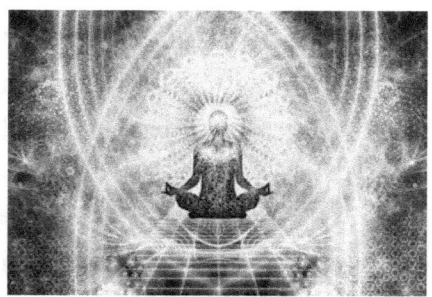

On the other hand, since Yoga is a practice known to the public for a longer time in the West, certain parts of the Tantric tradition are already well known and are used extensively to try to explain bioenergetic therapies. I refer specifically to the bioenergetic anatomy of the Chakras and the way in which they relate to our environment. Considering that this is a system already known to many people interested in one way or another in "bioenergetics", we will also refer to its bases in this manual.

We have added a small section in which we incorporate some notes about Japan's own bioenergetics. It is a scarce section, but it provides very revealing data about what Reiki really is and what we can expect from it.

I wish you to keep in mind that the knowledge that we will present in the basic bioenergetic chapter, although they can be applied to any aspect of life, does not strictly belong to Reiki techniques and its domain is not necessary to apply this healing system in an effective way. The reason that pushes them to incorporate them in this manual is that they offer us a global vision of the disease and provide us with a base from which to understand different concepts related to bioenergetics. These will help us better understand what Reiki is and how it acts. From this position, we can make use of the system with greater benefit and without falling into unclear conceptions or beliefs.

Unfortunately, many people, from their ignorance, trust the solution of all their problems to the practice of a technique (of Reiki or another type), without understanding that there is no real healing if there is no personal commitment to our health. It is not enough to know how to cook to eat properly. Similarly, it is not enough to start in Reiki to regain health.

With the concepts of basic bioenergetics and other knowledge added in the different parts that make up the manual, we intend to provide sufficient tools that allow the person who begins to practice the first level of Reiki to assume the task of enhancing their own health and that of those who are in charge.

Below are the basic foundations of the philosophies to which we have referred, as well as its relationship with Reiki, with special emphasis on the vision that health and disease offer each of these cultures.

Chapter 5: Research And General Acknowledgement

In the same way as other manifestations of back rub, shiatsu is generally accepted to have an unwinding impact on the body. There is additionally a lot of exploration recommending that pressure point massage strategies can ease sickness and heaving connected with a mixture of reasons, including pregnancy and soporifics and different medications. In one study, pressure point massage was demonstrated to essentially decrease the impacts of sickness in 12 of 16 ladies experiencing morning infection. Five days of this treatment additionally seemed to decrease tension and enhance inclination. An alternate examination, distributed in 1999, contemplated the impacts of pressure point massage on queasiness coming about because of the utilization of analgesics.

Reki Healing

Reiki is an otherworldly practice, now thought to be a type of pseudoscience, grew in nineteen twenty two by Japanese Buddhist Mikao Usui who has subsequent to been occupied by different instructors of differing customs. It utilizes a strategy usually called palm mending or involved recuperating as a manifestation of option pharmaceutical and is at times delegated oriental solution by some expert medicinal bodies. Through the utilization of this strategy, professionals accept that they are exchanging all inclusive vitality as qi with the help of the palms, which they accept takes into account recovering toward oneself and a condition of balance. These convictions have not been confirmed by cutting edge therapeutic science, and reiki has not been showed to be a compelling treatment for any perceived restorative condition.

There are ony two primary limbs of Reiki, normally alluded to as traditional Japanse reiki and the Western Reiki. Despite the fact that distinctions can be vast and changed between both limbs and conventions, the essential contrast is that the Westernized structures utilization systematized hand-positions instead of depending on a natural feeling of hand-positions (see underneath), which is usually utilized by Japanese Reiki extensions. Both extensions ordinarily have a 3 layered order of degrees, typically alluded to as the 1st, 2nd, and level of master, all of who are connected with against aptitudes and actions.

Reiki is taking into account a ki – an assumed life power which is simply speculative. Utilized as a therapeutic treatment, reiki presents no advantage:

the American Society of cancer, Research in cancer at UK, A national center for complementary and Alternative drugs have discovered no clinic or investigative source supporting arguments that Reiki is successful in the care of any sickness

Deduction of name

Mikao Usui (1865–1926)

Chujiro Hayashi (1880 - 1940)

English reiki or Reiki is a Japanese loanword reiki, which thusly, is a Chinese loanword língqì . The most punctual recorded English utilization day on 1975. Rather than the good transliteration, some English-dialect creator's pseudo-decipher reiki as "widespread life vitality".

Chinese língqì was initially listen in the Neiye "Internal Training" area of the Guanzi, portraying early Daoist reflection strategies. "That obscure crucial vitality inside the brain: One minute it arrives, the following it leaves. Its fine, there is nothing present inside it; so endless, there was nothing present the outside it. We lose it as a result of the damage brought on by mental unsettling." Modern Standard Chinese língqì is deciphered by Chinese-English lexicons as: " profound impact or atmosphere";["1. Brainpower; force of comprehension; 2. Heavenly power or constrain in children's stories; phenomenal power or power"; and "1. Profound impact ; 2. Cunning; shrewdness".

Beginnings

The arrangement of Reiki was produced by Mikao Usui in nineteen twenty two while acting
Isyu Guo, a 21 day Buddhist instructional class hung at "Mount Kurama"., however it doubtlessly included reflection, fasting, droning, and supplication to God. It is

asserted that by a mysterious disclosure, Usui had picked up the learning and profound force to apply and adjust others to what he was known as Reiki, he passed his body by his crown Chakra. In April 1922, Usui moved to Tokyo and established the Usui Reiki Ryōhō Gakkai and tried his best to keeping in mind the end goal to keep treating individuals on an extensive scale with Reiki.

As per the engraving on his dedication stone, Usui taught his arrangement of Reiki to more than 2000 individuals amid his lifetime, and sixteen of these understudies proceeded with their preparation to achieve the Shinpiden level, a level identical to the Western third, or Master/Teacher, degree. While showing Reiki in Fukuyama, Usui endured a stroke and kicked the bucket on 9 March 1926.

Early advancement

After Usui's demise, J. Ushida, an understudy of Usui, assumed control as president of the Gakkai. He was additionally in charge of making and raising Usui's remembrance stone and for guaranteeing the upkeep of the grave site. Ushida was trailed by Iichi Taketomi, Yoshiharu current successor to Usui, Kondo, who got to be president in 1998. Prior to Usui's demise, Chujiro Hayashi approached Usui about adding to an alternate manifestation of Reiki that was much easier. Usui agreed. After Usui's passing, Hayashi left the Usui Reiki Ryōhō Gakkai and shaped his own particular facility where he gave Reiki medications, taught, and adjusted individuals to Reiki, and it was to this center that Hawayo Takata was coordinated in the 1930s. Hayashi streamlined the Reiki teachings, focusing on physical recuperating and utilizing a more classified and less difficult set of Reiki systems

After Hawayo Takata got numerous Reiki sessions from Hayashi's trainees at his facility for diseases including stomach agony and asthma, Hayashi launched and prepared Takata to utilize Reiki, and she turned into a Reiki Master on 21 February 1938. Takata built a few Reiki facilities all through Hawaii, one of which was placed in Hilo and after that went ahead to go all through the United States, rehearsing Reiki and showing the starting level two levels to others and it was not before 1970 that Takata started starting Reiki Masters. At this stage, Takata likewise presented the term Reiki Master for the Shinpiden level. She focused on the significance of charging cash for Reiki medications and teachings, and altered a cost of $10,000 for

the Master preparing.

Takata passed on 11 December 1980, by which time she had prepared 22 Reiki aces, and pretty much all Reiki taught outside Japan can be credited to her work.

Usui's ideas and five standards

Usui was an admirer of the abstract works of the Emperor Meiji. While at present building up his Reiki framework, Usui abridged a percentage of the sovereign's works into a set of moral standards , which later got to be known as the Five Reiki Precepts . It is regular for some Reiki educators and professionals to comply with these five statutes.

Teachings

Reiki teachings guarantee that Reiki is endless and that it can be utilized to impel a mending impact. Professionals assert that anybody can get access to this vitality by method for an attunement procedure completed by a Reiki Master.

Reiki is depicted by followers as an all-encompassing treatment which realizes recuperating on physical, mental, passionate and profound levels. The conviction is that the vitality will course through the specialist's hands at whatever point the hands are set on, or held close to a potential beneficiary. A few teachings push the significance of the professional's proposition or vicinity in this procedure, while others assert that the vitality is drawn by the beneficiary's damage to enact or upgrade the regular recuperating processes. Further to this thought, the conviction is that the vitality is "canny", implying that the Reiki knows where to mend, regardless of the possibility that a specialist's hands are not display in the particular region.

Preparing

The instructing of Reiki outside of Japan is ordinarily partitioned into three levels,[68] or degrees, the most well-known of which are depicted underneath. Customary Japanese Reiki was taught seriously under Usui's direction, with week by week contemplation gatherings where Reiki was given and used to sweep the body so as to supply a fiery diagnosis,[69] which is referred to in Japanese as Byosen-hō, as a Japanese Reiki treatment is instinctive and particularly coordinated in examination to a Western Reiki treatment, which has a tendency to for the most part treat the entire body rather than particular ranges.

To start with degree

The main degree Reiki course, sometimes given the Japanese name of Sodden educates
 the fundamental hypotheses and methods. Various "attunements" are given to the understudy by the educator. Understudies learn hand situation positions on the beneficiary's body that

are thought to be most helpful for the procedure in an entire body treatment. Having finished the first degree course, Reiki experts can then treat themselves as well as other people with Reiki. Course span is subject to the Reiki Master Teacher; some hold four sessions spread more than various days, others hold two sessions more than two days.

Second degree

In the second degree Reiki course, now and then given the Japanese name of Okuden, the understudy takes in the utilization of various images that are said to improve the quality and separation over which Reiki can be applied. This includes the utilization of images to structure a makeshift association between the expert and the beneficiary, paying little heed to area and time, and after that to send the Reiki vitality. An alternate attunement is given, which is said to further build the limit for Reiki to move through the understudy, and in addition engaging the utilization of the symbols.[Having finished the second level, the understudy can work without being physically give the beneficiary — a practice known as "inaccessible recuperating".

Third degree

Through an exhaustive round of questioning, or "expert preparing", now and then given the Japanese name of Shinpiden , the understudy turns into a Reiki Master. In Reiki phrasing, the statement "expert" does not infer otherworldly illumination, and is infrequently changed to "Ace/Teacher" keeping in mind the end goal to keep away from this perplexity. As indicated by the particular limb of Reiki, either one or more attunements can be done and the understudy takes in a further image. Having finished the expert preparing, the new Reiki Master can adjust other individuals to Reiki and educate the three degrees. The term of the expert preparing can be anything from a day to a year or all the more, contingent upon the school and logic of the Reiki Master giving the preparation. There are usually two sorts of Master: Master Teacher and Master Practitioner; a Master Teacher is a Master of Reiki furthermore can show Reiki , however a Master Practitioner is a Master of Reiki yet does not instruct Reiki.

Varieties

There is much variety in preparing routines, rate of fruition , and expenses. Despite the fact that there is no accreditation or focal body for the Reiki, nor any of the practice , there exist associations inside the United Kingdom that look to institutionalize Reiki and Reiki practices, for example, the UK Reiki Federation and the Reiki Council (UK). Reiki courses are likewise accessible on the web, in spite of the fact that traditionalists express that attunement must be carried out in individual with a specific end goal to produce results, as the Reiki Master/Teacher doing the attunement must have the capacity to really touch the vitality field of the individual being adjusted. A separation Reiki attunement is not generally perceived by specific Reiki leagues, for example, with the UK "in-individual" or "up close and individual". Some people hold the perfect and good system that systems that look Reiki "rapidly" can't yield as solid an impact, on the grounds that there is not a viable replacement for experience and persistence when mastering Reiki.

At Western Reiki, it is mostly taught that Reiki lives up with expectations in conjunction with the whole meridian vitality lines and chakras through the utilization of the hand-positions of peoples, which typically relate to the 7th noteworthy chakras on a body. thats hand-positions can be used both on the front and back of the body, and can incorporate particular territories (see restricted treatment). As per creators, for example, James Deacon, Usui utilized just only 5 formal hand-positions, which concentrated on the head and the neck. when Reiki has been offered 1st to the head and then neck territory, particular regions of the body where uneven characters were available would then be treated. The utilization of the chakras is across the board inside Western Reiki, however not as much inside the Japanese Reiki, as it focuses all the most on treating particular zones of the body in the wake of utilizing strategies, for example, "Byosen-ho and Reiji-ho", which are utilized to discover territories of dis-simplicity in the emanations and external body.

Chapter 6: What Is Reiki?

This is the hardest question of them all. The simple answer is that...

Reiki is an ancient form of healing believed to have spread through Tibet, China and India. It was re-discovered in the late 19th century in Sanskrit teachings by Dr. Mikao Usui, a Japanese Christian minister and theology teacher. The word Reiki is Japanese, and means "Universal Life Energy", the same as the Chinese "Chi" or the Indian "Prana". Reiki is that vital life energy which flows through all living things and which can be activated for the purpose of healing to work on all levels - spiritual, physical, mental and emotional. Although it has its roots in ancient Buddhist teachings, Reiki is not a religion or a faith system. It is a healing system...

But this is just a dictionary definition. The following analogy is maybe a little more useful, though it is still limited. Imagine that you wake up in a strange room where all is darkness because heavy curtains or shutters cover the windows. Nature calls and you need to find the loo. You get out of bed and straight away you bump into a table, rattling the contents alarmingly and hurting your knee. Because of the darkness you have difficulty in finding your way around. The room seems huge and forbidding. Strange shapes loom out of the darkness as your imagination clicks in; too many late night movies and half remembered dreams. You are still in control but uncomfortable and the pressure in your bladder is making itself felt. You need to find the light switch. After a bit more crashing about you find it and switch on the light. That simple action changes everything - you can see. You quickly find the door, switch on other lights and do what must be done. You recognize the dark shapes for what they are and when you check your clock you see it is later than you imagined and on opening the shutters you are greeted by a bright, shiny morning. All you did was push down on a small piece of plastic and things changed in an amazing way. You did not need to know how electricity was generated or how electricity works. All you needed to know was that to get light you push down on the switch. Someone had done all the hard work before you. If you feel the need then by all means research electricity but it won't make the light come on any faster or better. Simply knowing how to use the light is what counts, then making the most of it. To do this there are a few things you need to know; that there is a lighting system in the first place and what to do if it seems not to be working and who to contact. If you had never seen an electric light before you would need to be shown these things but once shown it would not be long before you were switching lights on and off with the best of them. You might at first think it was all magic but as you know it is not the sort of magic that can be done any better by special people or by those who wear special clothes and sing special songs. Anyone can switch on a light if they want to. Switching on the light is easy. Then what you can do in the light is endless on the other hand you can remain as you are and sit in the dark. The choice is always yours. Think of Reiki as that switch. It allows you to see what is wrong, who you are, what you can do and how to do it. Seeing all this is just the start. What you do then, is your choice.

Chapter 7: Reiki's Negative Side

Synopsis

As with anything in life, there are always good and bad sides. Reiki proves to be no different. Making the decision to embark on the process of acquiring reiki skills takes time and effort. A certain amount of commitment and perseverance is expected which is sometimes difficult to muster in this "instant gratification" expectations of today's society.

What To Watch For

To ensure the potential reiki practitioner is able to garner positive energy, certain sacrifices needs to be made. Refraining from consuming meat, fowl or fish a few days before attempting a reiki session is a prerequisite.

As purity is the ultimate goal when practicing reiki, consuming food and drink items that contain drug, pesticides, toxins and other negative ingredients are strongly forbidden. These negative elements cause the body system to be thrown off balance and so disrupting the smooth flow of positive energy.

Going on a water of just juice fast is encouraged. Minimizing caffeine intake or cutting it out altogether is also required. These elements also create imbalance in the nervous and endocrine system. Other things to avoid at least three days before practicing a reiki session are alcohol, sweets, and smoking.

Keeping a quiet and peaceful lifestyle is also encouraged, however this may prove to be difficult in the fast pace surroundings of everyday life. Reducing exposure to outside negative elements is also necessary, thus watching TV, listening to unsettling music and reading distressing news are all discouraged.

Keeping away from all other negative mental states, like, anger, fear, jealousy, hate, worry are important, as these emotions can block a person from achieving a successful reiki session.

In some extreme cases, reiki practitioners tend to ostracize themselves from others, simply because they consider those around them "contaminated" and full of negative energy, which they don't want to be connected to.

Chapter 8: Is Reiki Vitality Recuperating Craftsmanship A True Blue Practice?

The National Center for Complementary and Alternative Medicine perceives Reiki as a manifestation of vitality pharmaceutical deserving of extra study. Specialists might want to have the capacity to clarify 'how it lives up to expectations", on the grounds that there is little question that it "does work" for some individuals. Albeit there may even now be pundits, since there dependably are, the vast majority n the medicinal services callings now acknowledge the authenticity of Reiki.

It is equivalent to chiropractic consideration and needle therapy, however not as predominant. In view of the way of Reiki vitality mending workmanship, it can be utilized by back rub specialists, medical attendants and other guardians. It doesn't require broad or extravagant direction. Specialists have recommended it as an integral procedure for different professionals.

Individuals are so usual with Reiki back rub, and maybe now consider of it as one unmistakable system. Reiki is totally unique in relation to back rub treatment, however it is very commonplace to see them blended into one methodology. Reiki demonstrates, widespread life power, and that really talks about the extremely base and importance of what it is precisely about. Really, the same indistinguishable components that can be found in Eastern combative technique and even yoga are additionally fundamental in Reiki. Only one rule which encapsulates the seven chakras of the human body are a fundamental piece of the Reiki knead method. The premise for wellbeing with this and different treatments and techniques is in light of the solid dissemination of life supporting vitality in the body.

What Reiki treatment will do is add to finish cool and peace all through the body so strain is discharged. So it is anything but difficult to perceive why Reiki is regularly coupled with back rub treatment so the chakras can get to be more open and solid. At the point when the body is satisfactorily casual and can legitimately adapt to regular anxiety, then that will bring about a more prominent energy to mend itself. It is no puzzle that a solid body has the capacity safeguarding itself and supporting a sound and solid condition of being. One vital standard of Reiki mending involves the idea of accomplishing offset. After advancement has been made, then we must work to keep our vitality stream adjusted at all times.

Western pharmaceutical has since a long time ago distinguished the part of an excess of anxiety and the inability to manage it as forerunners to numerous diseases. Another view on that, which is the Eastern idea, is an individual's life and general body are not in an all around adjusted state. Regularly you will find numerous outer viewpoints, for example, terrible eating and extra poor decisions that just compound the condition. Reiki and back rub are every now and again utilized to bring the body into a more casual state. Rubbing essential ranges of the body will help the body to alleviate stress.

We might want to discuss Reiki alongside needle therapy on the grounds that there are significant examinations. Each of the two systems are concerned with empowering the flow of life power, of vitality, in the body. Likewise, both of these regions are in light of the idea that physical and mental issues happen because of a blockage or confinement of the characteristic development of our life power, or vitality, inside our bodies. We are helpless against ailment, wellbeing issues or passionate issue as indicated by where the vitality confinement is occurring. Simply think about all the different negative sorts of deduction and conviction that people may have. We should have a few illustrations, and they are touchiness, nerves, frightfulness, misery, disappointment, and so forth.

The force of joining Reiki vitality remedial mending in addition to body back rub is regularly extremely powerful for some individuals. At the same time, we ought to say that, characteristically, you will need to be willing to consider the standards of this general comprehensive methodology. Yet, it is helpful to note that Reiki back rub has gotten to be broadly acknowledged in Western nations. Reiki remedial back rub is about a vital methodology which proposes you ought to utilize it on-going in your general quest for wellbeing.

Lately Reiki has ended up surely understood as an option mending method and has been generally honed. The principal vital thing to know and comprehend is that Reiki, or some other option treatment ought to never take the spot of treatment and exhortation of an authorized restorative specialist or professional. Reiki, then again, can be a powerful complimentary treatment that can upgrade your consistent therapeutic treatment.

A Reiki treatment session starts all that much like a back rub treatment session. You can hope to be in a private room or zone and the Reiki treatment will be performed while you lie on a back rub table. You will be requested that wear baggy open to dress and to evacuate gems. You will have a sheet or cover for spread and be offered pads to guarantee your solace. The expert ought to have unwinding reflection sort music playing and there may be incense or some type of fragrant healing being utilized.

The expert will request that consent touch you. In the event that you are not open to being touched, make sure to tell your specialist as Reiki is pretty much as successful without touch.

The expert will then do an output of your body to get a vibe for your vitality and where you may have issues that need vitality mending work. The output is finished by basically moving the hands over the entire body without touch. The specialist will presumably make inquiries while doing the sweep. Correspondence with your expert is imperative; don't be modest about interfacing with your specialist.

After the sweep the treatment will start. The specialist will put their hands tenderly on your head or shoulders. Reiki is a light touch treatment so the touch will be exceptionally tender with insignificant weight. The professional will travel through the treatment hand positions until they have secured your whole body. Amid your treatment your expert may blow on you or give a sharp hand applaud. This is by and large done when attempting to evacuate a blockage and is a piece of the treatment process.

It is imperative to realize that a Reiki professional ought to never touch you straightforwardly in any private zone. On the off chance that this happens you ought to leave the session as the specialist is not carrying on in an expert or satisfactory way.

While getting your treatment you will start to feel warm and loose. Numerous individuals enter a light contemplation state. You may encounter a mixed bag of sensations amid your treatment. You may see hues, feel shivering sensations, experience serious feeling, have flashback recollections, smell distinctive fragrances, or any mix of tactile observations. Convey what you experience to your professional.

After your treatment lie still the length of you have to. Try not to attempt to get up too quick the same number of customers feel inebriated for a little time. You might likewise feel tipsy, woozy or exceptionally euphoric. Unwind and take as much time as required.

Amid the week or something like that after your treatment you may experience a detoxification. Reiki will discharge blocked energies on all levels of your being and any physical blockages discharged need to be killed from your body. You may have side effects of regurgitating, loose bowels, second rate fever, sweats, or different indications. This is ordinary after a Reiki treatment, yet in the event that it endures for more than a day see your doctor as there may be another restorative condition bringing about the indications.

Reiki chips away at all levels of being, physical, mental, enthusiastic and otherworldly. The Reiki vitality goes to any region required and starts the mending methodology. You may require more than one session to perform the mending required. I am certain that you will need more medications as a Reiki treatment is such a positive and euphoric experience.

Chapter 9: The Sacral Chakra

The Sacral Chakra is the center which senses power. It connects you with your feelings and allows you to live in the now. It is also closely linked to your joy, happiness, and enthusiasm. If you want to be in tune with this chakra center then you must review issues like your emotional stability. You must determine if you are in control of your true feeling or if you are just pushing them back into hiding so you don't have to feel them. Furthermore, you must know if his inner child is uninhibited, enthusiastic, and alive. It is important that you review your created perception to find out if it's restricted or if you are open minded and able to think freely outside of the box.

A person who has a strong Sacral Chakra is person who has respectful and mutual sexual relationships. They aren't limited by impotence or frigidity, and they are comfortable with their partner.

If you want to boost the power of your Sacral Chakra and encourage the flow of orange energy, you can embrace sensation. You can take advantage of deep tissue massage, hot aromatic baths, and water aerobics. You can take cooking classes and watch emotional movies. You are also encouraged to consume orange foods and drinks. Furthermore, aromatherapy oils like tangerine, neroli, mandarin, orange, and Melissa can be used. Flowing or bouncing music can boost this chakra. Orange stones like Carnelian or Coral can be worn or carried. Since orange is the color of the Sacral Chakra, I encourage you to use it in art, bath, décor, and clothing.

The Sanskrit name of the Sacral Chakra is Svadisthana and it is located in the lower abdomen area, below the navel. It deals with intimacy and social issues and connects with your sensing abilities. If this chakra is not balanced, it's possible you may suffer from eating disorders, depression, allergies, asthma, low back pain, yeast and Candida infections, drug and alcohol abuse, sensuality issues, frigidity, impotency, and urinary problems. To stimulate the chakra center, you can engage in water aerobics, embracing sensation, hot aromatic baths, and massage. You can also eat and drink orange-colored foods and liquids. Orange essential oils are also good for your body as well as wearing orange clothing and gems.

The Sacral Chakra relates to the lumbar plexus, sexual organs, and reproduction system. Its endocrine gland is the gonads. It is concerned with sex and food and aims to satisfy the body's needs and wants. It relates to your desire to have children. If the Sacral Chakra is balanced, you can communicate, listen, and respond appropriately to your needs and wants. If there are tensions, this chakra will reflect in your consciousness regarding your emotions or will in connection to what your body is longing for.

The Sacral Chakra deals with your sexuality and feelings and if it is opened, the feeling is released and expressed without being too emotional. If you have an open Sacral Chakra you will be passionate, outgoing, and open to affinity. You will have no problems with your sexuality. If this chakra is under-active, you can be impassive or unemotional and closed to people around you. If it is overactive, you can become emotional and sensitive all the time. Furthermore, this will allow you to be very sexual and comfortable with your sexuality.

To open the Sacral Chakra, you must sit on your knees, relaxed and with your back straight. You then lay your hands on your lap with your palms on top of one another and facing up. The left palm must be underneath and must touch the right hand's back fingers. The thumbs must also touch gently. Next concentrate on the meaning of Sacral Chakra then chant "VAM" in a silent yet clear manner. You must be relaxed while thinking about this chakra and how it affects your life. The routine must be repeated until you feel completely relaxed.

Chapter 10: Additional Reiki Protection And Cleansing

This chapter has additional techniques for protection and energy cleansing, taken from different schools of Reiki and healing.

Why is protection and cleansing important? It is important because we need to make sure we are working with positive energy, and that we are able to remove any negative or unwanted energy. For example, if you feel like you have picked up on a client's energies after or during the treatment e.g. a physical symptom or any negative emotions.

You don't have to use all of these techniques – just focus on one or two and use the rest for reference. These techniques are mainly just for the healer only (you don't want to scare your client).

Your teacher should teach you about protection and cleansing. You should be able to contact your teacher (or any other good teacher) if you have any questions or concerns.

ARCHANGEL MICHAEL

One of the most popular ways to protect yourself is to use Archangel Michael, the angel of protection. This can be done by prayer or visualization e.g. "Archangel Michael, please protect me, and my client."

CHOPPING/DECORDING

After a healing treatment, you want to make sure that you have not absorbed anybody else's energy. For this reason, you can do chopping/decording.

Simple make a chopping action with your hands around your body, starting with your head, all the way down your body, back, legs and feet. Clap hands and stamp feet afterwards to ground yourself.

ADDITIONAL INFORMATION FOR ADVANCED STUDENTS

BUBBLE OF PROTECTION

Another common way to protect yourself (energy, spiritually, emotionally) is to imagine a bubble of protection around you. You could imagine a cloak instead, or a zip from your feet to your head, which you zip up to protect yourself.

GOLDEN EGG

A similar method is the Golden Egg. Imagine pure white light energy flowing into your crown chakra and filling your body. It nows flows out of your body, into your aura, forming a Golden Egg of protection.

SALT BATH OR COLD SHOWER

You can also cleanse yourself of spiritual, emotional, mental and physical energies, by having either a cold shower, or a hot bath. Whilst doing this you can scrub yourself gently with sea salt, or just say a prayer ("May this water cleanse me.")

CRYSTALS

Some people use certain types of crystals for protection and/or cleansing e.g. clear quartz.

HERBS AND AROMATHERAPY

Another method is using a smudge stick, white sage, incense or frankincense to cleanse and protect. These are available from health shops or the internet.

To cleanse your body, start with the top of your head and waft or wave the white sage / stick / scent down (never upwards) around all of your body and aura. To cleanse a room, waft or wave the white sage / stick / scent in every corner of the room and also the centre of the room.

CRYSTAL CAVE SYMBOL

In Tibetan Reiki, a Crystal Cave symbol can be used for protection. You could find out more information for a training course.

CLOSING DOWN & CLEANSING

You can also do a mini closing down meditation after the healing. This is a protection meditation.

-   Sit or lie down, make sure your back is straight.

-   RELAX: Gently breathe in and out. Maybe count after every out breath. If you can, use diaphragm breathing, as this is more relaxing and helps your parasympathetic nervous system.

- CLEANSE: Imagine yourself at a beautiful lake, waterfall or paddling in the sea.

- Imagine that you are using this water to cleanse and purify your whole body, including your aura. Let the water wash away any negativity from you.

- Step out of the pool.

- CLOSE DOWN: Now imagine that there is a giant zip from the bottom of your body to the crown of your head. You are going to now zip up your body from your feet, to your head (do front and back). Do once or repeat if you like.

- This zip has now closed, forming a protector bubble or cloak around you.

- Gently start to come back to being fully awake.

- If you are deeply relaxed, start to wiggle your fingers and toes, and then gently open your eyes.

Maybe have a glass of water. Sit until you are ready to carry on with your day (rather than getting up too quickly).

GROUNDING (can be used on clients)

If you or your client feel lightheaded for a while after the Reiki treatment, its a good idea to "ground" yourself. The purpose of this is to focus your energy back down to earth, as you are too high up. This can be as simple as going in the garden, watering the houseplants, being around nature.

You can also do a grounding meditation: make sure your back is straight when you meditate. Breathe in and out and imagine yourself being surrounded by nature. Imagine there are roots growing out of your feet into the centre of the earth. Do this for the amount of time you feel is necessary, long or short, and then come back, opening your eyes.

Another method for grounding is simple breathing in and out (maybe sit or a chair whilst you do this). Then place one hand on the floor and imagine your energy connecting with the ground and the earth. Imagine that all the negative energy is flowing into this ground. When you feel ready, finish and say thank you.

SPECIAL CIRCUMSTANCES

Occasionally, when working with energy, you can come into trouble if you are not trained properly, experienced or are using bad practice. This is why a good teacher is needed.

If you find yourself having disturbing experiences e.g. spiritual, then contact your teacher, or any good Reiki teacher.

You also need to be careful that you don't rush your Reiki training or spiritual practice as you may find it too powerful, too quickly. This has have consequences on your health and wellbeing. If you are following traditionally Reiki schools, it is better if you leave at least a few months in-between each Reiki level.

JAPANESE SELF-CLEANSING

(for the healer, not for client)

PRINCIPLES/PRECEPTS

Another way to protect and cleanse yourself is to say the principles out loud or to yourself. Do this whilst in Gassho position (hands in prayer position in front of chest).

BRUSHING OR DRY BATHING (KENYOKU)

There are different versions of this. Here is a popular one (thought to be the original Usui method):

A Gassho (hands in prayer position in front of chest) should be done at beginning and end of this practice.

Quickly move your right hand (flat position, fingers together) from left shoulder diagonally down to right hip, whilst exhaling, saying "ha". Do this fast and in a straight line.

Quickly move your left hand (flat position, fingers together) from right shoulder diagonally down to left hip, whilst exhaling, saying "ha". Do this fast and in a straight line.

Repeat steps 2 and 3 at least once.

Quickly move your right hand (flat position, fingers together) from left shoulder down arm to your left fingers. Do this fast and in a straight line. Exhale at the same time.

Quickly move your left hand (flat position, fingers together) from right shoulder down arm to your right fingers. Do this fast and in a straight line. Exhale at the same time.

Repeat steps 5 and 6 at least once.

Raise your hands in the air, palms facing together in prayer but shoulder width apart. Visualise yourself connect with the Reiki energy, which flows in to your hands and through your body.

Sit with hands on lap facing upwards. Make sure your back is straight. Breathe through nose and focus on your breath running through your body. Imagine a white light going through all your chakras.

Now imagine this white light expanding from your chakras into the whole of your body, and then your aura.

Put hands in prayer position in the centre of the chest (heart chakra). Make sure your back is straight. Imagine you are breathing through your hands. Inhale and imagine that the white light is running into your hands, your chakras and whole body, filling you with energy, love and positivity. Exhale and imagine that the white light is coming out your body again, taking away any negativity. Repeat as many times as you like.

Sit quietly and relax. Say thank you for the energy and white light. If you would, you can finish off by saying the Reiki principles.

BREATHING TO CLEANSE (JOSHIN KOKYUU-HO)

This is to cleanse your spirit. A version of this is also used in martial arts, such as Tai Chi.

Sit or lie down, making sure that your back is straight.

You are just going to breathe in through your nose, and out through your mouth.

As you breathe in, imagine the Reiki energy coming in through your crown chakra, all the way down your body, into your stomach (near your naval chakra). This is the energy centre known as your Hara or Tanden.

Hold the breath and let the energy spread throughout this area and your whole body.

Now breathe out and imagine this energy coming back out of your body into the ground through your fingers, hands, feet and toes.

Repeat as many times as you like.

Finish and say thank you in prayer (Gassho) position.

REIKI SHOWER

Sit, stand or lie down (back must be straight). Close your eyes and relax.

Put your hands in a prayer position at the centre of your chest (heart chakra) and do a Reiki dedication (i.e. asking for Reiki to be sent to cleanse you). If you're attuned, you can use Reiki symbols and mantras.

Put your hands above your head, shoulder width apart, palms facing down. Imagine Reiki energy going from your palms to your whole body and aura. This energy is cleansing you.

Gently move your hands down over your face and body (not touching but at a distance). All the time, imagine the energy is flowing from your hands to your body and aura, then feet, cleansing you.

Palms now face the floor. Imagine all the negative energy is coming out of your palms and your feet, into the ground.

Sit quietly with hands in prayer position in front of chest (heart chakra). Say end dedication (thank you and close down).

SELF-PURIFICATION (JIKO JOKA HO)

This is the same as Hado Kokyo Ho but in a standing position (see chapter on Japanese Techniques).

Different sounds are associated with healing different types of the body. The most famous is "om" which is the Universal sound and heals on every level. This meditation uses the sound "haa" which is associated with the immune system and blood. For more sounds and their associated healing, see "The Barefoot Doctor: Liberation".

Stand with feet apart and knees slightly bent. Make sure your back straight and eyes closed,

Say prayer or Gassho Gassho.

Breathe in and out through your nose.

STAGE 1: Still in prayer position, raise your hands up above your head, but with a distance between the hands. Channel Reiki through your hands.

STAGE 2: When you start to feel this energy flowing down into your body, bring your arms out to the side with palms facing down.

STAGE 3: With your palms still facing down, place your hands in front of your chest with fingertips touching (so that your hands form a straight line parallel to the ground).

STAGE 4: Breathe out saying "haa" for as long as you can, whilst pushing the hands towards the ground. Don't force the breath, keep it natural.

STAGE 5: Breathe in and move hands to forehead, still palms facing down.

STAGE 6: Breathe out saying "haa" whilst moving hands down with palms facing the body.

Repeat as many times as you like.

Say thank you in prayer (Gassho) position.

Chapter 11: Creating The Atmosphere For Workshops/Attuning

One of the beauties of Reiki energy is the sense of connection it gives with others, the planet, and the community of Reiki healers all over the world. This is the new energy that is emerging. In order that we all feel it and that you pass it on to your students, we suggest you include a homage to the Circle of Reiki Healers and an invitation to join this circle in your workshops. This enables students to tune in to the pool of energy awaiting them with Reiki. Several elements are important in the creation of the circle.

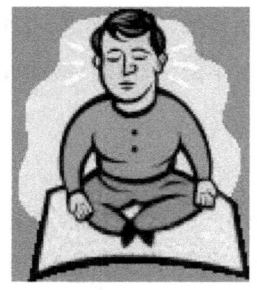

Beauty

Include an altar in your classroom honouring the Reiki Masters that guide you. Include symbols of anything meaningful to you, pictures etc.

Meditative Space

Utilise music, incense, light, chanting both before the session and during the work, if this feels appropriate. Teaching people how to meditate, breathe, open up and ground is practical and useful.

Guided Meditations

Use the Circles Meditation, others suggested or one of your own that acknowledges the Earth, the lineage of the Reiki Healers, the students and other appropriate elements. We encourage you to bring into this part of the class that which is most meaningful to your own progression. People resonate with the space that YOU create more than techniques.

The Council Format

Use the talking stick principle or a similar device to allow people to share from the heart, without interruption, about their process and their experiences with Reiki. Just being heard without judgement is a gift and very much in keeping with the Reiki principles.

Safety

Make sure that everyone feels granted permission to share the sometimes vulnerable and personal feelings that come up in the attunements. Assuring people of confidentiality, compassion, etc. is important. Allow all, not just yourself, space and time to express themselves fully.

Comfort

Practicalities are important. Make sure there are enough comfort breaks. No one can concentrate if they need the loo! There will be changes in body temperature for many. Be prepared to accommodate this. Take care of yourself also.

Enjoyment

For all concerned is a priority. Allow it to come in with humour.

Accepting and Celebrating Oneself as a Healer

The most difficult and also the most rewarding aspect of teaching Reiki is that people are amazed to see themselves as healers. The attunements give people the opportunity reclaim their birthright. This can be a very moving experience for most. They say that they are home, that they always knew this was part of their soul's purpose etc. The recognition of oneself as healer can be a very tender and fragile moment. It is important that they have the space to accept this as part of their self-definition. You can be very affirming at this time.

Encouragement of practice, praise for taking the step, heartfelt acknowledgement of the heat and power in their hands - these are all important elements in anchoring the experience for people. Too often, we have heard that people have attended a Reiki workshop and felt that nothing happened. It is part of our job to allow people to make meaning and sense of the experience in the context of their own life's story.

Ask people to remember when they felt their healing potentials, whether that be in childhood or later in life. A guided meditation to this effect can always be helpful. Having practice partners give feedback about warm hands or sensitive touch can bring the natural healer out more fully in a person.

Perhaps the most immediate result people have with Reiki is in *self-healing.* Always give people the homework of completing Reiki sessions on themselves before they come to the second day. When the healing warmth and comfort of a Reiki session in bed before sleeping and arising is firmly anchored in one's experience, the practice is well begun. A sister Reiki teacher describes herself as a "horizontal mystic". She uses Reiki each morning combined with breathing practices as her meditation. What seems to be true is that one develops a "relationship" with Reiki.

The more time and practice one devotes, the greater the energy becomes.

Our planet needs more healers. Each person who takes on the joyful task of being a conscious healer enriches their individual life and the collective life of the earth. We have a tremendous opportunity to gently usher many souls into the healing way. A healer in every home soon?

Let's do it now.

Circles

These can be used for starting or finishing a group session.

The Circle's rules are simple and powerful. Circles will be your main tool for gaining information, feedback and taking the "pulse" of the class. One way to keep the circle on target is to state the question(s) you want answered, such as "What is one valuable thing you learned today that you are going to put to use?" Setting an overall question helps everyone keep their focus on the purpose of the circle. Use the circle to help create a sense of equality for all of the participants. Below are principles underlying circles.

1. Ask who would like to share first and go around in a circle from that first speaker. Allow people to "pass", but always come back to them after everyone else has spoken, or when they ask to speak. **You** can share after everyone else has done. It is okay if some still choose to not share.

2. Acknowledge each person in turn both at the beginning and end of their comments. Check the time with each, allowing space to express themselves but also gently keeping them to the point.

3. Acknowledge each person with "Thank you". If you use any other phrase,

such as "That's good", or "Very interesting", be prepared to compliment everyone in a like manner. Try to be unbiased about the views expressed.

4. The one absolute rule is do not allow anyone to speak out of turn or intrude upon someone else's sharing. If someone does this, politely stop them and let them know you will get to them soon.

5. A talking stick avoids interruption. This can be any object which can be passed around easily. The principle is that folk only speak when they are holding it.

6. For **opening** circles, objects such as love balls can be used to assist in bonding. These can be soft type balls [velvet is good] which are filled with love and tossed across the circle, calling the recipient's name as it is passed. This can be developed by the giver adding words such as: Hope, Peace, Clarity, Trust or similar

uplifting expressions. This is great for bonding with a new group

7. If it is a **closing** circle linking together for sending love and good thoughts out into the universe is often the intent. Each person may choose a word which is their feeling for the day. Angel / Blessing cards or similar are useful expressions of good thoughts. This builds up the feeling of positive energy within the circle. Raising hands in the air to launch the love into the atmosphere finishes it off well. Give thanks and rest.

8. Sharing Reiki HUGS is an acknowledged finish.

Chapter 12: The History Of Reiki

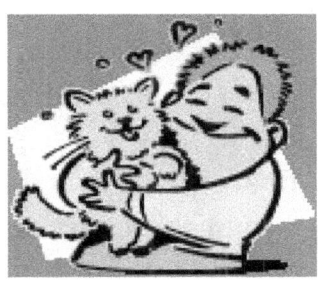

DR. USUI'S REIKI: REDISCOVERED REDEFINED

There has been much controversy in the last several years regarding the traditional Western version of Reiki's history. It seems that parts of the story provided by the former "Grand Master," Mrs. Takata, has been sensationalized. The version passed down to me specifically states, "This is the history of Reiki as it was handed down to us by Mrs. Takata." It concludes with,

"Some of the story has been found to be untrue."

I am including elements of Reiki's origins that have kept repeating throughout my research. With great interest, I have perused more than several "traditional" accounts. Apparently, certain facts have been either diminished or exaggerated to make it more palatable for those with Christian backgrounds and the more conservative. Therefore, new information pertaining to the origins of Reiki as previously practiced in Japan has been very eagerly welcome. However, as the telling of Reiki's history is important, the traditional story of Reiki, regardless of its unverified facts, is unique and part of the Reiki culture.

There are two main segments to Dr. Usui's Reiki. One originated in the West (the traditional story) as verbally passed on by Mrs. Hawayo K. Takata to her students, beginning in the 1930s. The Eastern story is from Japan (found on his Japanese memorial tombstone) where this form of Reiki began.

The Usui System of Natural Healing has evolved over time. In its current state, it is much more organized and structured than the simple, flexible, intuitive method practiced by Dr. Usui. Following is the Western description of the Usui System of Reiki.

THE TRADITIONAL WESTERN STORY

Dr. Mikao Usui was born on Aug. 15, 1865 in Japan. He was raised by Christian missionaries and studied the Bible and teachings of Jesus. At that time, most children were raised

There are two main segments to Dr. Usui's Reiki: the Western traditional version and the Eastern Japanese story.

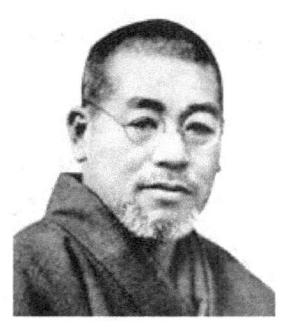

Dr. Mikao Usui

Dr. Usui astutely contemplated passages in the sutras and each time gained deeper insights.

under the traditional Shinto and Buddhism religions. He studied religion, which led him to become a professor of theology. This religious training led him to become the minister of a Christian boy's school in Kyoto, Japan. During his appointment, he continued to be enthralled by the healing abilities of Jesus and the Bible. One day, some students asked him about the healing methods used by Jesus Christ and if he believed in them. He answered with an assured yes. They continued to question him as to whether he would be able to carry out such a healing for them. Dr. Usui was stunned and unable to answer these questions. This set him to ponder many things. He soon resigned his position and his search began, determined to find the answers of this mystery.

As Christianity was not popular in Japan, Dr. Usui journeyed to America. He spent seven years studying the scriptures. He was not satisfied and no closer to finding the truth. He also studied the teachings of Buddha, his disciples, and accounts of healings. They seemed similar to his studies relating to Jesus. Further discoveries between Christianity and Buddhism led him back home.

Upon returning to Kyoto, Japan, Dr. Usui went to live at a Buddhist monastery. He meditated and began studying Sanskrit (one of the oldest languages) formulas and symbols in old Buddhist sutras (scriptures). In the interim, he befriended the head Zen Buddhist abbot at this monastery, who greatly inspired him. Dr. Usui's inner gifts and healing awareness continued to expand.

During the next several years, Dr. Usui astutely contemplated passages in the sutras and each time gained deeper insights. He seemed closer to the answers he sought. His tenacity expanded and deepened his self-awareness. He realized how great was the mind in its ability to create and heal physical, emotional, and mental illnesses. He was now ready to receive additional knowledge, which were very close at hand and bring his work to completion.

Dr. Usui decided to seek refuge at a sacred Buddhist mountain retreat near Kyoto. This area had special healing energy, a high level of life force energy. Before departing, he asked the abbot to collect his remains for burial should he not return after 21 days. Dr. Usui's intention was to fast and meditate during these three weeks (21 days) in the hope of: 1) gaining contact with the level of consciousness the Sanskrit symbols had been written with, and 2) helping others by determining the truth of the symbols' contents.

As he walked the 17 miles to Mt. Kurama, he noticed a tranquil spot next to a stream and waterfall. (Some accounts relate that Dr. Usui stood under the sacred waterfall to gain healing and clarity.) He came to a spot facing east and gathered 21 stones to use as a calendar, marking each day. Each day he cast one stone to keep track of passing time. During his meditations, his concentration was very strong and his vibrational field quite pure. He was able to experience his own inner light and purity.

The 21st day left him with one stone. He knew his quest was reaching an end. At dawn, he saw a bright moving light in the sky. It began moving very rapidly toward him. He stood there as it became bigger and brighter until the light struck his forehead and he went into a trance. He was in a euphoric state, envisioning many colored rainbow bubbles. Soon they changed into white glowing bubbles. Contained within each bubble was a three-dimensional Sanskrit character in gold. Dr. Usui said, "Yes, I remember." On a deeper level within, he knew the essence of these symbols—pure love, wisdom, compassion and bliss.

Dr. Mikao Usui now had the wisdom and healing knowledge as did Buddha and Jesus. As he walked down the mountain with this realization, he experienced what is traditionally known as four miracles.

The Four Miracles And Birth of a Healing System

First, he stubbed his toe walking. His palms turned hot and he placed his hand on the injury, quickly healing it.

Secondly, he reached an inn at the foot of the mountains. He ordered a full meal of cold rice and cold tea – not the wisest choice for breaking a long fast. However, he ate it without any discomfort.

Dr. Usui's primary focus was for the improvement of

body and soul.

Third, the servant girl at the inn was nursing a bad toothache. Dr. Usui took notice and placed his palms on her jaw, healing her pain.

The fourth miracle took place at the monastery in Kyoto. Dr. Usui returned to find his friend the abbot in bed with arthritis. Once again, through the placing of his hands on the abbot's body, another healing took place.

Dr. Usui was guided to take the method into the slums of Kyoto. He lived there for several years doing healings on the town beggars. After healing many, he asked his patients to start a new life. However, many returned to the streets to beg once again. Dr. Usui became discouraged to find those he physically healed still begging instead of making an honest living. Many of the beggars were angry their physical bodies had been healed, which no longer would allow them to make their "earnings" as beggars. These free healings only addressed the physical and ignored their minds and spirits.

Additionally, Dr. Usui became quite popular after a horrendous earthquake near Tokyo. He helped survivors with great success and his reputation soon spread.

Through interacting with individuals from all walks of life, Dr. Usui discovered two very important factors:
1. A person should ask for healing.

To be more effective, he introduced four symbols for focusing the healing intent. They continue to

be part of The Usui System of Natural Healing as "the four symbols of Reiki."

2. There should be an exchange of energy for the healer's time- an exchange of energy.

It is worthwhile to note that Dr. Usui's primary focus was for the improvement of body and soul. Self-healing was an integral part of this system. To be more effective, he introduced four "keys," or symbols, for focusing the healing intent. They continue to be part of **The Usui System of Natural Healing,** passed down to students and known as "the four symbols of Reiki."

Chujiro Hayashi

Dr. Usui began to teach Reiki throughout Japan. During his travels, he gained clarity as to the purpose of the symbols he experienced during his mountain retreat. He used them to attune people so they could become teachers and travel with him. It was at this time he met Chujiro Hayashi, a retired naval officer still on reserve status. Hayashi received his Reiki Master's training from Usui in 1925 and became Usui's successor. Usui attuned 16 or 18 men and women — including 16 Masters — in his lifetime.

Hayashi opened the Shina No Machi healing clinic in Tokyo, where healers worked in groups on people who lived there during the healing process. Hayashi trained teams of Reiki practitioners, including Hawayo Takata, the next important figure in the Reiki story, who arrived at the clinic for healing.

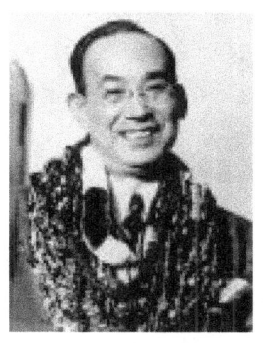

Chujiro Hayashi

Hawayo Takata

Mrs. Takata was a resident of Hawaii. She was ill with a diseased gall bladder and decided to visit her family in Japan and take care of her health. Her condition did not improve so she resorted to surgery.

The night before the operation, she heard a voice tell her, "The operation is not necessary."

She went against her intuition and continued with the surgery proceedings. On the operating table, while being prepared for the anesthetic, she asked the surgeon if there was another way for her to heal. The doctor told her of Hayashi's clinic and she was taken there the next day.

Takata lived at the clinic and was completely healed in body, mind and spirit in four months. She asked to be trained in Reiki. She was refused at first because Hayashi was not in favor of Reiki leaving Japan at that time. Eventually he relented and Takata received her Reiki I training in Spring 1936. She joined the teams of healers at the clinic and received her Reiki II in 1937. After living in Japan for two years, Takata returned to Hawaii.

In 1938, Hayashi visited Takata in Hawaii where they went on a lecture tour together. It was at this time, Feb. 22, 1938, that Takata received her Mastership from Hayashi. He announced that Takata was to be his successor and instructed her not to give Reiki attunements away without charge. He also told her when he summoned her, she was to go to Japan immediately. In 1941, Takata awoke one morning to see a vision of Hayashi standing at the foot of her bed. She knew this was the summons that she was expecting, and took the next available boat to Japan.

When she arrived at the clinic in Japan, Hayashi and other Reiki Masters were present. He announced there was a great war coming and the clinic would be closed. He was concerned Reiki would be lost altogether, and therefore, wanted a foreigner, Takata, to be his successor. Hayashi knew he would be called to service since he was a Naval reserve officer and he decided to accept his own death instead. On May 10, 1941, in the presence of his students, Chujiro Hayashi stopped his own heart from beating and died. The war he predicted was World War II. The clinic was taken over during the occupation and Reiki was no longer available in Japan.

Takata was the means by which Reiki survived. She brought it to Hawaii, then to the United States mainland, and finally to Canada and Europe. Many times she would train members of the families of the seriously ill if they were not strong enough to participate in the trainings. Her students were not allowed to take notes, and her instruction on healing positions varied from time to time. The trainings themselves were not identical from student to student, which may account for the variations in Reiki treatments today. She trained hundreds of people and designated 21 Reiki Masters in the West before her death at age 80 on Dec. 11, 1980.

Dr. Usui wholeheartedly held a vision of a profound
awakening within one's heart, which is termed as honu no reiko.

Aligning With Dr. Usui's Intentions

Each Reiki practitioner is aligned with the energy and circumstances surrounding Reiki. Dr. Usui wholeheartedly held a vision of a profound awakening within one's heart, which is termed as **honu no reiko**. He held this intention for each person to whom he taught and gave attunements. Dr. Usui's memorial inscription provides deeper insight and clarity into his original intentions. It is for this reason that I have included the inscription written on his memorial stone in Japan. The text below is by the author and translator, Frank Arjava Petter and his wife Chetna M. Kobayashi.

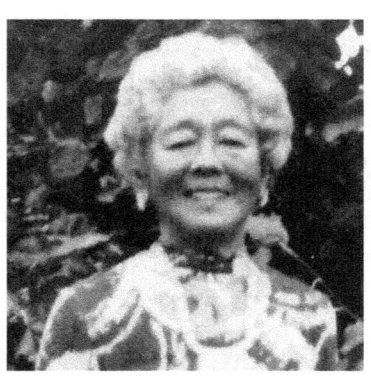

Hawayo   **Takata**
THE EASTERN VERSION

Memorial Inscription: A Moving Translation

The following information is taken from the inscription on the Usui Memorial dating from 1927, and was written in old Japanese by Mr. Okata, a member of the

Usui Reiki Ryoho Gakkai, and Mr. Ushida, who succeeded Usui-Sensei as president of the society.

The large kanji at the top of the 10 x 4-foot memorial stone reads: "Memorial of Usui-Sensei's Virtue." The remainder of the inscription reads as follows:

"Someone who studies hard (i.e. meditation) and works assiduously to body and mind for the sake of becoming a better person is called a man of great spirit. People who use that great spirit for a social purpose, that is, to teach the right way to many people and to do collective good, are called teachers. Dr. Usui was one such teacher. He taught the Reiki of the universe (universal energy). Countless people asked him to teach them the great way or Reiki and to heal them.

"Dr. Usui was born in the first year of the Keio period, called Keio Gunnen, on August 15th (1865). His first name was

Mikao and his other name was pronounced either Gyoho or Kyoho. He was born in the village of Yago (Taniai) in the Yamagata district of Gifu prefecture. His ancestor's name was Tsunetane Chiba. His father's name was Uzaemon. His mother's family name was Kaweai. From what is known, he was a talented and hard working student. As an adult, he traveled to several Western countries and to China to study, worked arduously, but at one point, did run into some bad luck. However, he did not give up and trained himself arduously.

One day, he went to Mount Kurama on a twentyone day retreat to fast and meditate. At the end of this period, he suddenly felt the great Reiki energy at the top of his head, which led to the Reiki healing system. He first used Reiki on himself, then practices improve tried it on his family. Since it worked well for various ailments, he decided to share this knowledge with the public at large. He opened a clinic in Harajuku, Aoyama, Tokyo in April of the 11th year of the Taisho period (1922). He not only gave treatments to countless patients, some of whom had come from far and wide, but he also hosted workshops to spread his knowledge. In September of the twelfth year of the Taisho period (1923), the devastating earthquake shook Tokyo. Thousands were killed, injured, or became sick in its aftermath. Dr. Usui grieved for his people, but he also took Reiki to the devastated city and used its healing powers on the surviving victims. His clinic soon became too small to handle the throng of patients, so in February of the 14th year of the Taisho period (1925), he built a new one outside Tokyo in Nakano.

His fame spread quickly all over Japan, and invitations to distant towns and villages started coming in. Once he went to Kure, another time to Hiroshima prefecture, then to Saga prefecture and Fukuyama. It was during his stay in Fukuyama that he was hit by a fatal stroke on March 9th, of the fifteenth year of the Taisho period (1926). He was 62 years of age.

Dr. Usui had a wife named Sadako; her maiden name was Suzuki. They had a son and a daughter. The son, Fuji Usui, took over the family business after Dr. Usui's passing.

Dr. Usui was a very warm, simple and humble person. He was physically healthy and well proportioned. He never showed off and always had a smile on his face; he was also very courageous in the face of adversity. He was, at the same time, a very cautious person. His talents were many. He liked to read, and psychology, fortune

religions around the world was vast. This lifelong habit of studying and gathering information certainly helped pave the way to perceiving and understanding Reiki. Reiki not only heals, but also amplifies innate abilities, balances the spirit, makes the body healthy, and thus helps to achieve happiness.
his knowledge

telling, and of medicine, theology of To teach this to others, you should follow the five principles of the Meiji Emperor and contemplate them in your heart. They should be spoken daily, once in the morning and once in the evening:

1. Don't be angry today.
2. Don't worry today.
3. Be grateful today.
4. Work hard today (meditative practice).
5. Be kind to others today.

The ultimate goal is to understand the ancient secret method for gaining happiness (Reiki) and thereby discover an all-purpose cure for many ailments. If these principles are followed, you will achieve the great, tranquil mind of the ancient sages. To begin spreading the Reiki system, it is important to start from a place close to you (yourself), don't start from something distant such as philosophy or logic.

Sit still in silence every morning and every evening with your hands folded in the "Gassho" or "Namaste" position. Follow the great principles, and be clean and quiet. Work on your heart and do this from the quiet space inside you. Anyone can access Reiki, because it begins within yourself.

Philosophical paradigms are changing the world. If Reiki can be spread throughout the world, it will touch the human heart and the morals of society. It will be helpful for many people, not only healing disease, but the Earth as a whole. Over 2,000 people learned Reiki from Dr. Usui. Even more learned from his senior disciples, who carried Reiki further. Now, after Dr. Usui's passing, Reiki will continue to spread far and wide. It is a universal blessing to have received Reiki from Dr. Usui, and to be able to pass it on to others. Many of Dr. Ususi's students converged to build this memorial here at Saihoji Temple in the Toyotomi district.

I was asked to write these words to help keep his great work alive. I deeply appreciate his work and I would like to say to all of his disciples that I am honored to have been chosen for this task. May many understand what a great service Dr. Usui did for the world".

Work on your heart and do this from the quiet space inside you. Anyone can access Reiki, because it begins within yourself.

Chapter 13: Reiki Treatment Method - The Most Powerful Spiritual Healing Arts Yet Very Smooth And Healthy

Reiki healing is perhaps the most smooth and satisfying method of healing individuals, but within this soothing and relaxing program, an extremely potent healing strategy is actually at work.

This unique form of therapy offers you a number of benefits. The most important and foremost is stress relief. With reiki you can enter a deep relaxation condition utilizing mind-calming exercises. This meditation as well as relaxation techniques have been shown to be a highly effective stress reduction technique. Many of the physical health conditions that people have originated with psychological stress and anxiety from existing events around them, and from their past as well.

Reiki will work together harmoniously with current day medicine. Reiki therapy may be employed on just about anyone, irregardless of their faiths and perceptions. Religion and faith usually do not affect reiki treatment whatsoever, even if the religious practitioner or subjects are experiencing some type of 'close to god' emotion, still, reiki is good for all people.

Reiki therapy can be a bit different for one person to the other. For example, some therapist have to touch their patients but some just need to hover their hands somewhat above the individuals system. Often the reiki restorative healing session begins with generating a relaxed condition for the patients. They have to loosen up with ease on a chair or on a massage therapy table, and then the therapist begins the particular healing process, by starting their aura after which they situate their hands over the person's body and generally stay there for a while before shifting positions.

Could depend on the individual's body region which is the focus of the problem, the hand positions may likely stay on just one area all throughout the healing period or in a different spot, and last as long as necessary for the universal energies to transfer through the chakras. During the reiki healing period of time, the individual should feel relaxed and happy and quite often the individual becomes drowsy or actually falls asleep throughout the session.

Reiki Remote Healing - 3 Methods of Achieving Reiki Healing Over Distance

As you may now know Reiki Healing is an ancient Japanese art of healing performed by the placing of hands over a person - thereby directing or transmitting a healing energy to the body, or specific area of the body, which may be effected by illness.

Reiki Remote Healing or Reiki Distance Healing

The Reiki Master does not need to be in close proximity to the recipient, for the healing effects of Reiki to work. In fact they could be a Continent apart. Many people have reported significant results both physically and emotionally - most feeling the effects, or energy, almost immediately after the Remote Healing session has started.

3 Methods of achieving Reiki Remote Healing

Obviously if the person is separated from the Reiki Master then the tradition laying of hands is out of the question. However, there are number of ways in which the energy can be transmitted to the patient instead.

1. Intention. By this method the Reiki Master visualises his or her body as that of

the recipients, then by placing their hands over their own body, they can transfer the healing energy to the same body area of the patient. This requires a certain level of concentration and is considered to be used by more experienced healers.

2. Symbols. This method is used whereby a Healer uses a symbol or object, to help focus the energy to the recipient. This can take the form of a photograph or drawing of the patient, which is used as a focus. Alternatively, focus can be achieved by use of a proxy in the form of a doll or teddy bear. Even a pillow can be used for that purpose.

3. Crystals. Using Crystals for healing is a whole subject in itself. When used for Remote Healing the Reiki Master prepares the Crystal or stone to transmit the energy to the person he or she is treating. Once the correct Crystal or stone has been selected, the Master focuses their

Intention on the object, thereby using it as a conduit to send the healing energy it accesses.

Become A Reiki Healer

Are you looking in becoming a Reiki master?

Have you looked all over for different ways in gaining experience and certification, but can't figure out the best way?

Let me explain to you what it takes to become a great Reiki master as well as show you the best program to help you become a pro in this art of healing.

Three degrees of Reiki

Reiki is an ancient art of healing through the use of energy. It can be learned, taught, and practiced in different degrees.

These degrees are divided into three categories, with each one at a higher level than the other.

These three degrees are simply referred to as: first, second, and third.

First Degree allows you to focus on teaching a student everything that they have to know about the art of energy healing.

In this degree you will be taught what Reiki really means and what it can do for you.

Masters will give their students in-depth descriptions about Reiki which will include where it came from, the proper way of using it, and how to give it.

After all concepts are taught, hands-on practice will then take place.

After completing the first degree of training, a student will know how to use energy for self-healing.

All of this energy can also be channeled to help others, as well as stimulate personal and spiritual growth.

After learning this first degree, you will be able to expand and elevate your emotional, spiritual, physical, and mental state.

The second degree starts to lead you into a deeper understanding of the ancient method of Reiki healing.

Here you will be introduced to the sacred symbols which you can use to develop your awareness of healing others, your self, and helping with the lives of others.

The flow of energy within you intensifies.

You will be able to enhance your abilities through the symbols as well.

Distance healing then becomes taught, and is possible at this stage.

With distance healing, you can learn to heal another person even if they are miles away.

In the third degree of training, it can sometimes be divided into two subgroups.

The first group is where you become a master and are capable of teaching other students.

The second group is focused on the improvement of yourself only.

Third degree is mostly for those who wish to further develop themselves into becoming a Reiki master.

You will have access to all the symbols and are able to perform attunement on others.

There are also more complex healing cycles taught at this level, which aim in expanding your knowledge and experience.

The end goal here is to make you a master in this art, where you can initiate, train, and teach others.

Remember this, Reiki is not a 'quick' subject that you can learn in a couple hours. It requires a calm mind.

Chapter 14: The Fifth Chakra

The fifth chakra is located in the throat, and it deals with truth and falsehood. It is blocked by denial and the lies we tell ourselves out of shame or guilt. The fifth chakra is called *visuddha* in Sanskrit, and is thought to open our minds to the astral bodies, the inner worlds, and the realization that we weave our reality with the power of our thoughts and words. It is also more commonly called as the sound chakra.

The sound chakra

The sound chakra focuses on our need for communication, and our ability to express ourselves through words and verbal cues. Understand that sound itself is an energy, and because we live in a world of sounds, it is important to filter them- to learn how discern the truth from the lies. It is equally important that we avoid spreading lies ourselves, as these falsehoods are sources of negative energy, confusion and misunderstanding. The lies we tell ourselves and others, block the sound chakra's ability to recharge and help you speak and seek the truth. The more the sound chakra is blocked, the easier it is to become confused and lost in this world of multiple truths and beliefs.

Opening the sound chakra

Follow the simple steps below to open, cleanse and recharge your sound chakra.

Step 1: Stand or sit cross-legged under the blue sky. The fifth chakra resonates strongly with all things blue, and so being under the sky for a few minutes every day gives your sound chakra a boost.

Step 2: Hum a familiar, simple tune as you prepare yourself for deeper communication with yourself.

Step 3: As you hum, think of all the times you have denied yourself. What lies have you tried to tell yourself about your identity, your abilities, your strengths and your weaknesses? Remember that you cannot lie to yourself, because deep inside you will know when you speak the truth.

Step 4: Now, think of all the times you have lied to others, or denied them their identity, rights and opportunities to improve. Why did you allow falsehood to come out of your mouth? Were you afraid or jealous?

Step 5: Take a deep breath, and release all of the denials and falsehoods you have uttered or thought. Surrender them to the universe, to the great expanse of blue sky above you. Release them, and know that the truth inside you is stronger than the lies you tell yourself. Release them and understand that you will only be truly happy if you envelop yourself with truth.

You can also recharge your fifth chakra by drinking any pure liquid such as water or fruit juice in general, and by eating lemons, limes and grapefruits in particular.

Chapter 15: Yoga For Health Problems

Yoga practiced continuously and sincerely helps in curing and recovering from almost all types of health problems. It is a boon in our life to solve the health complications with little effort. Here are the few regular problems which one face in our day to day life.

Headache

Uttanasana (Standing forward bend)

Stand straight in mountain pose keeping feet close to each other. Then bend down from hips, lightly bending the knees keeping the torso on the legs. Now keep the hands straight next to your leg. Looking straight slowly inhale and expand your chest to stretch your spine. While exhaling, press both the legs straight. Try keeping the knees as straight as much as possible.

Shshu asana (Child pose)

Sit on your heels and slowly bring your torso forward and make the head rest on the ground with your hands in front of you, parallel to each other. Now press your chest on your knees by lowering it. Hold for a while and relax to normal position.

Back pain

Dhanurasana (Bow pose)

Lie down on stomach head facing the ground, keeping both legs close and toes straight. Now bend the legs as much as possible towards hip. Now hold both the legs tightly and exhale. Now while inhaling, raise your chest above and head stretched up. It gives a curvy shape to the body, allowing it to stretch in all directions.

Bhujangasana (Cobra pose)

Lie down on your stomach with your head facing the ground, keeping both legs close and toes straight. Now keep the palms on ground beneath shoulders near to your torso. Let the hands be parallel to each other. Inhale and lift your head then chest and abdomen. Stretch to an extent where navel touches the ground. Now with the help of your hands (putting equal pressure on both) pull back the torso. Stay a while and breathe for the air to pass through all the curves.

Stress management and depression

Bhujangasana, Uttanasana, Januhasasana are few of the many yoga poses to be performed to manage stress and depression. It is all about bringing calmness and giving peace for a while where we tend to forget what our situation is.

Blood pressure

Pashchimottanasana (Posterior stretch pose)

Sit with leg extended forward. Keep legs a little apart, straight and toes pointed upward. Lifting the torso by the sides, extend forward towards your toe with hands straight, fingers close and pointed. Bend forwards without bending the knees and hold the feet with hand (fingers around the feet).

Halasana (Plow pose)

This is a complex posture helping in stretching the spine and hip. Lie down flat on the back with legs straight and hands by the side palms facing down. While inhaling lift the legs up there by lifting hips straight up with hands on the ground and torso at a 90 degree angle. Now move the leg slowly and touch the floor with toes. Press the hands tightly on the floors.

Digestive problem

Bhujangasana, makarasana, trikonasana are some of the many yoga postures which we can practice for curing digestion problem. Apart from that we can also do -

Veerasana (warrior pose)

Stand straight with legs close by and hands by the body side. Stretch left leg forward from right leg to the maximum possible distance. Now bend the knee to 90 degree angle and exhaling keep both hands on the knee with hands joined by palms. Now inhale and raise the closed hand up above your head and look at the celling. Stretch the hand backwards to the maximum possible extends thereby bending the spine. Hold a while and breathe normally. It gives a curved position to look at.

Menstrual problem

Matsyasana (fish pose)

This pose gives a stretch on the thyroid gland thereby reducing the blood flows to the legs. The reproductory system is improved as this increases the blood flow.

To start with, take supine position and cross one leg on the other (ideally take "padmasana" i.e. keep the foot of one leg on the other legs thigh). Now bend backward by stretching the elbows up and pushing chest and head forward. Keep the head on the ground slowly with neck bent backward giving an arch like pose. Bring back the hands and touch the toes of the leg with opposite hands, i.e. left hand touching right toe and vice versa. Take a minute's time and breathe normally keeping the eyes closed.

The other asana that can be practiced are Halasan, veerasana, dhanurasana, Paschimottanasan.

Chapter 16: What Is Illness?

Illness is a manifestation of unbalance. It manifests in the energy field first and if the cause of this unbalance is not corrected, it will start to manifest in the physical body at some point in time. It might start as a mild pain. As times goes on, and if nothing is done to address the cause, the pain or discomfort might get stronger and stronger. Until eventually it becomes a disease. Again that disease can get worse and become chronic, if the energy is not balanced and the flow of energy is not restored.

Most people just want to get rid of symptoms. We stop a headache with a pill. We stop a cold with some medicine. But one way to look at it is that all illnesses are psychosomatic. What does this mean? Psychosomatic does not mean that it is not real, or that you do it on purpose to get attention. What it means is that it has been created by the mind. When I explain to people that all illness is psychosomatic they usually cringe at the thought they are responsible for it, but I find it incredibly empowering. It is the same part of your mind that ensures that all goes well in your body (the blood pressure, the heart rate, etc) that can also create the problems. Why does it do it? It is a way for the brain to tell you what needs to be corrected. Illness is a language. It tells you what needs to be put right in your life, your diet or your body. If you don't get enough sleep for example, there is no point drinking lots of coffee. You need to address the cause. And if it is stress then do a life review to see if you can remove the cause of stress or find better ways to deal with it.

Consider how often illnesses are metaphors: "he is doing my head in" might create a migraine. You can have neck pain literally because someone is being a "pain in the neck" to you. Many books have been written about this and psychologists have made extensive studies on the subject. There is no shame about having psycho-somatic illnesses, because as I explained earlier, most illnesses are psychosomatic. This means in turn that if you take responsibility for it instead of blaming fate or others, then you can restore your own health. Sometimes we are stuck in situations that make us unhappy and we can't see how to get out of them, but this is what is needed to heal. I would recommend **Louise Hay's book, You can heal your life,** for a good introduction to this link between mind and body.

Sometimes too, an illness can talk about a family setting or a relationship, as I have seen people take on other people's problems very often. This is particularly the case for children.

What is healing?

Reiki is a transfer of pure energy that is channelled through the giver to a willing recipient. You will notice that I did not add that reiki brings results. It is not given with the intent to cure. Why? I guess we go back here to the notion of karma. We have all contracted our lives and the events that it brings to us. Who is to know if the illness wasn't willingly contracted as a lesson for that person and should we "cure" them we would deprive them of an important life lesson. Just to get back to what I was explaining in the previous chapter, if illness is our friend and is here to tell us something, masking the symptoms does not help the person get better. It only postpones the problem.

Reiki is just pure energy that the recipient receives and uses for her best interests. Does that mean that if they are not meant to heal then it's not worth bothering?

Well, the healing energy we send might help them understand the root of the problem. It might help them cope better with what is happening to them. That can already be a huge improvement in their lives.

Is the death of a client a failure for a healer? I don't believe so. The failure would actually be the fact that you stopped giving them healing because you think they are going to die. The role of the healer is to respectfully send unconditional love to their clients, regardless of their situations. This also means that if that person's time has come to die, then the healer should be there every step of the way to support her – unless of course the healer doesn't feel she is capable of it, in which case it is important to refer the person to another person. If we are dealing with our own issues around death and are not clear then it's best not to help others lest we will project our problems into them. There is something very beautiful in being able to accept nature's transition and to help someone get to the other side peacefully. Your healing might help that person be more comfortable in her last hours, it might help her feel supported and peaceful.

I would conclude this chapter by saying that I believe healing is not curing. Healing is just to give some love to someone who needs it to get them through their illnesses, regardless of the outcome.

Why people don't heal?

Sometimes we wonder why some people who come to us don't seem to get better. There can be several reasons for this state of affairs.

As we mentioned earlier, it could be that they actually have to go through this illness to learn a lesson and that they cannot step out of it until the lesson is understood.

It could also be that they have "contracted" this illness to be a way out of this earth as an experience. This is meant to be what ends their existence on this planet. Their time has come.

But there are also a lot of cases, where people who come to you actually don't want to heal. They might vehemently deny it or claim that if only they could get better, then they would be happy. However the truth is that however painful or debilitating their condition might be, they will not let it go. Why is that?

First because what people fear most is change, above anything. And this fear does not depend on whether change is positive or negative. We are creatures of habit and any change in our lives is stressful.

Secondly, sometimes their illness has become their raison d'être. They identify with the illness so much that they have become the illness. How many people say they are cardiac instead of saying they have a heart condition? Or that they are asthmatic instead of saying that they have asthmatic crisis. The difference is huge. The first step in healing is to distance yourself from the illness yet accepting it wholly and not try to fight it but embrace it to learn its lesson. When do you get your asthma attacks? After you have an argument with your partner? When you go to work? Aha. Do they realise that just because they have had asthmatic episodes does not mean they will be asthmatic for life. But if all their friends have the same condition and if they get attention from it, it can be very frightening to open up to the idea of letting go of the condition. It is also quite hard to separate oneself from one's ailments because the way western medicine sees us is only as carriers of illness. There is no holistic approach and as a result a lot of "patients" become their condition.

Thirdly, they might subconsciously be scared of being well again. Suddenly it would deprive them of a lot of the attention or support that they get and they wonder how would they cope on their own. There is for example the retired woman who has a heart attack and suddenly her children and grand children come and visit her, whereas before, she was visited much less often. If she got better, would it really improve her life? She might prefer to be unwell but surrounded by her loved ones. So in reality, she has a lot to lose if she gets better. Our role as "healers" is to show her that she can get that attention in different ways.

Lastly they might believe that they are not able to change and that to be well means to be lonely. Some people have been told by their doctors that their condition is not curable or that there is nothing that can be done about it and it becomes a self fulfilling prophecy. And although as healers, it would be irresponsible to promise any results, it is important to show people that nothing is impossible. There are sufficient cases, documented for example, by **Bernie Siegel** in his admirable book "**Love, Medicine and Miracles**", to show that patients often prove doctors wrong. At least those doctors that accept to be amazed and don't discard the "spontaneous remission" cases as something that they can't explain so it is not true.

Change, even for the better, is considered by everyone as something quite stressful. Most of us prefer our painful current existence to jumping into a void of the unknown, even if someone promises to us that it will be better. Firstly, how do we know that they are right and that it will actually be better? This thought often stops us from trying a different approach.

But also, very often our relationships are weaved around our current patterns and changing might mean that we lose our friends and even our loved ones. It might also mean seeing less of our families if they are not willing to support the new "us". This reminds me of when I quit smoking and I realised that the people who I thought were my friends nearly didn't comment on it and even in some cases tried to sabotage my efforts. It took me some time to realise that it was because they secretly wanted to quit but didn't have the courage to do so, and as a result resented me. This is such a common response. The same happens, if you want to loose weight, if you want to move from an unhappy relationship to a happy one, and so on and so forth. You might find that you outgrow your friends. And that can be scary. So sometimes, people stay the same to keep their support system, however unsupportive. They prefer that rather than face the risk of being on their own. To them, bad company is better than none.

Chapter 17: Chakras

The word Chakra is derived from the Sanskrit word meaning "wheel", "circle" or "cycle" but perhaps even a better translation would be spinning wheel. As it symbolizes movement from one dimension to another, it is referred as a "chakra," or "wheel", although practically it is actually a triangle.

Chakra - 'Energy & information exchanging center between physical body & etheric body'.

Chakra is actually a term which defines a number of lines meeting on a common specific point.

What is the chakra system?

In Hinduism, chakra is thought to be an energy point or node in the subtle body. Chakras are believed to be part of the subtle body, not the physical body and as such, there are the meeting points of the subtle (non-physical) energy channels called Nadi.

Each chakra is responsible for delivering energy and information to specific parts of the body. When they are blocked the body becomes sick and the flow of energy is diluted. A full Reiki healing re-opens the chakras and re-balances the flow of the universal life force energy around the body.

According to ancient Vedic texts, there are many chakras in human physical and etheric body but 7 chakras play a major role. Hence these 7 chakras are called as the "Major chakras". Major chakras are located along the spine extending out from front and back of the physical body; they regulate the flow of life force energy into our physical bodies. We also have a number of minor chakras in our body.

The chakras we are talking about are both physical & metaphysical. In the physical body, these chakras are a result of the intersection of various nerves or Nadi's which form major & minor energy meridians that carry the energy to different parts of our body. In metaphysical terms these chakras are a result of the intersection of our Nadi's in our subtle bodies.

The position of each chakra is in correspondence to our endocrine glands that are responsible for the release of hormones in our body. Every chakra corresponds to a specific aspect of human behavior and development. Chakras empower us to maintain balance on the physical, mental and spiritual level. They differ in size, energy and activity from person to person. Each chakra has a particular sound, color, which vibrate to a particular frequency. Each chakra needs to be balanced and energized properly.

How does chakra influence on your Physical, Mental and Emotional wellbeing

Physically - each chakra is associated with certain part/organ of the body. It transforms the energy and information the organs need to function effectively.

Emotionally - chakras signify specific aspects of human behavior and growth/maturity.

Mentally - they vibrate at different levels relative to the awareness and ability of the individual to receive intuition.

Functions of chakras:

From bottom:

☐ Muladhara Chakra /Root Chakra - element Earth

It is located at bottom of the spinal column; it is also called as Kundalini. It is the base from where 3 Nadi's emerge (Ida, Pingala & Sushumna). Muladhara is the foundation of physical energy & wellbeing.

The root chakra/base chakra is the primary chakra of our body which acts as an energy pathway and connects us to our physical body and the Earth. The root chakra is associated with the color red which represents passion, strength and fire.

Functions of the Root Chakra

Physical

Physically, it is responsible for the proper functioning of the legs, feet, bladder, kidney and spine. It keeps us nourished and healthy, also states good financial condition or growth, promotions and Earthly pleasures.

An imbalanced root chakra can cause several problems such as fatigue, hemorrhoids, arthritis, constipation, lower back pain, weight issues, immunity problems, frequent illness, depression, eating disorders, skin problems and diarrhea. It can also cause sleep disorders or financial loss.

Emotional

When the root chakra is balanced, you feel confident and gain respect and trust. You will face any critical situation or conflict with a calm and constructive mind.

When it is imbalanced you will feel tired, overly cautious and insecure. Fear surrounds you; any task seems difficult which results in violent aggressive behavior, anxiety, laziness, obesity, overeating, instability and materialistic.

You might also get "stiff", anxious and become narrow minded.

Addictions

Gambling, food, work, shopping.

Spiritual

This chakra mainly focuses on **Survival**, if balanced; it meets all the basic needs of life such as food, shelter, warmth and comfort. "**Trust**" is the key to clear any blockages related to Root chakra. Release the "**Fear**" so you can trust the flow of life. Trust that the life supports you in every possible way for your overall upliftment.

Exercising and walking supports to clear blocks related to Muladhara chakra.

☐ Swadhisthana Chakra/Sacral Chakra - element water

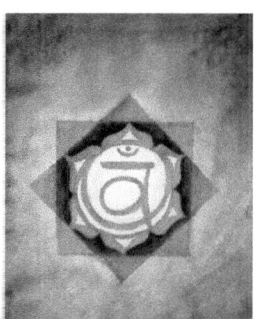

It is located just below the navel. It is connected with the sense of taste (Tongue) & reproductive system (Genitals). This is the energy center for creating relationships of all kind.

The swadhisthana is the second chakra. It deals with feelings and expression of emotions. The sacral chakra is situated in the lower abdomen about 1-2 inches below the navel. The swadhisthana chakra is associated with the color orange which represents honor and power.

Functions of the Swadhisthana /Sacral Chakra

Physical

This chakra is responsible for the proper functioning of the reproductive system as well as administrates lymphatic, circulatory/ cardiovascular system and the urinary tract. As the sacral chakra mainly deals with purification, the chakra plays a major role in removing toxins from the body.

An imbalanced swadhisthana chakra can cause physical issues such as urinary problems, kidney stones, lower back pain, gynecological problem and prostate problems. It controls sexual organs, reproductive system, bladder and the kidneys.

Emotional

If balanced it promotes positive emotions such as; joy, ambition, love, healthy relationships and creativity. You feel more comfortable in expressing your emotions and feelings. You naturally give and receive love, affection, with no guilt or shame. It expands knowledge and breaks boundaries makes you feel comfortable around people and work towards your passion.

If this chakra is blocked then you suppress your emotions/feelings, you turn out to be shy, helpless and weak. Blocks in this chakra can also lead to jealousy, seductive manipulation, and addiction to pleasure, sensitive and strong emotions, revenge and lack of creativity, depression, pressurizing, obsessive attachment, emotional dependency or may lead to suppress someone knowingly.

Addictions

Laziness, alcohol, sex, smoking.

Spiritual

This chakra mainly focuses on **Pleasure**, if balanced; it promotes healthy relationships, emotional intelligence and ability to change. "**Forgiving and loving yourself**" is the key to clear any blockages related to sacral chakra. Release the "**Guilt**" it just punishes you and creates pain. Learn from the past and move on positively.

Gardening, cooking, taking care or playing with pets/children supports to clear blocks related to swadhisthana chakra.

☐ Manipura Chakra/Solar Plexus Chakra - element fire

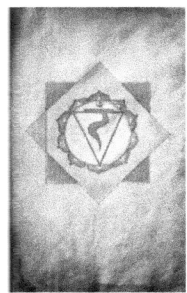

It is located at the center of the body, just above the navel. It helps in digestion process & also develops willpower & energy level in the body.

The Manipura chakra is the third chakra in the chakra system. The Manipura chakra is associated with the color yellow which represents strength. The solar plexus chakra or Manipura is also known as "the diamond", as it is the center of the energy. It is called the solar plexus chakra because of its location being close to the solar nerve plexus.

Functions of the Manipura / Solar plexus Chakra

Physical

This chakra administers every organ in the body that produces energy and participates in the purification process. This chakra manages the autonomic nervous system, stomach, gall bladder, large intestine, liver and pancreas, whole digestive and muscular system, cellular, respiration system and even the eyes are governed by the Manipura chakra.

Issues with the digestive system, arthritis, diabetes and hypoglycemia are some physical problems connected to the imbalance of this chakra. You may feel tiredness, body aches and laziness too.

Emotions

When the chakra is in balance, you feel confident, enthusiastic, calm, cheerful, expressive and flexible. You handle any difficult situation with peace of mind. Cheerfulness, joy and spontaneity will be your basic nature. Intuition flows easily at the right time, life feels completely balanced, you will be sensitive to others feelings and spread love and compassion towards all.

If this chakra is imbalanced; anger, depression, frustration, dominating-controlling behavior, isolation, doubts and aggressiveness surrounds you. Lack of interest in any activity, inability to work hard, lack of concern, bad habits and fear of being controlled by others keeps you isolated. Sometimes this may even result in arrogance, manipulative, power hungry, stubbornness, hyperactivity, excessively ambitious and competitive nature.

Addictions

Cocaine, drugs, alcohol, over diet, work and anger.

Spiritual

This chakra mainly focuses on **willpower**, if balanced; it promotes good mental and physical strength. "**Focusing on your inner-power**" is the key to clear any blockages related to manipura chakra. Release the feeling of "**Disgrace**" *(*Shame**)** feel good about yourself. Be open for healing.

Exercising, swimming, running, deep meditation, helps to clear blocks related to manipura chakra.

☐ Anahata Chakra/Heart Chakra - element air

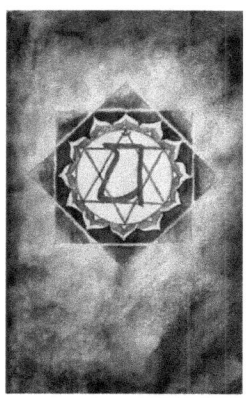

It is located near the heart & gives us the ability to express love. It connects to the sense of touch & actions. Anahata promotes the ability to make decisions based on one's higher self (following your heart) which can manipulate the chain of Karma.

The heart or Anahata chakra is the fourth chakra of the seven main chakras. The Anahata chakra is associated with the color green which represents unconditional love.

Functions of the Heart Chakra

Physical

The heart chakra administrates the lungs, heart and blood circulation. It is also associated with the thymus gland which is essential for a healthy immune system.

When this chakra is blocked, you may face health issues such as breathing difficulties, high blood pressure, lung diseases, breast cancer, heart attack, pain in shoulders and arms, upper back etc.

Emotions

If this chakra is balanced one easily develops self-love and love towards all and will be happy and easy going. Positive changes occur in relationship or friendships.

When this chakra is imbalanced one may face emotional ups and downs, divorce, separation, emotional abuse, isolation, abandonment, feeling of rejection and grief due to death. It also raises emotions such as possessiveness, resistance towards love, overly sacrificing and paranoid feelings.

Addictions

Drugs, ego, sugar, conditional love, overeating, physical abuse, bad language.

Spiritual

This chakra mainly focuses on **Love**, if balanced; it promotes good and happy bonding. "**Understanding**" is the key to clear any blockages related to Anahata chakra. Release "**Grief**", a person or the relationship has served its part in your life, let-go it with love. Meet new people and spread happiness.

Being compassionate, learning to forgive and spreading unconditional love helps to clear blockages related to heart chakra.

☐　Vishuddha Chakra/Throat Chakra

It is positioned at the throat region. Vishuddha is associated with creativity, communication & hearing. It produces hormones essential for growth & clears malnutrition. Vishuddha is associated with genuineness/truth.

The Vishuddha Chakra is the fifth chakra associated with the color blue which represents purification. It is related to the ears and mouth due to its association with hearing and speaking respectively.

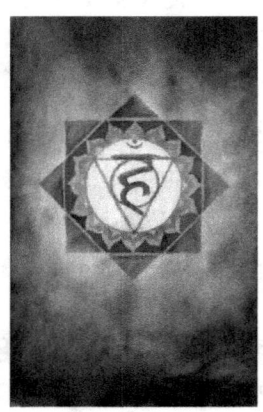

Functions of the Throat Chakra

Physical

Physically, this chakra is associated with the thyroid gland and the endocrine system. The thyroid gland plays a vital role in releasing hormones that are important for growth and development. It regulates the body's metabolic system and is responsible for the proper functioning of the ears, nose, teeth, mouth and throat.

When the throat chakra is blocked, it may cause physical defects such as laryngitis, chronic throat defects, hypothyroidism, fatigue, hoarse voice, cold sores, jaw pains, gum defects, headaches and obstruction in speech.

Emotions

The throat chakra is connected to self-expression, listening and communication. When this chakra is balanced, we listen to people and respond in a proper way. We develop good listening skills, pleasant voice, and clear communication, ability to hear and speak truth.

When the chakra is blocked communication is harmed. You may lie, interrupt and gossip unnecessarily. Excessive talkativeness, harsh words make you lose your value. You may even develop anger, hatred and bitterness.

Addictions

Harsh words, tobacco, bruxism (teeth grinding), lies.

Spiritual

This chakra mainly focuses on **Truth**, if balanced; you words are valued. "**Self-expression**" is the key to clear any blockages related to Throat chakra. Avoid "**Lies**" it damages relationships. One lie turns all truth into questions. Make people understand the situation instead of lying. Understanding brings peace.

Practising silence, singing, chanting helps in clearing blocks of vishuddha Chakra.

☐   Ajna Chakra/Third Eye Chakra

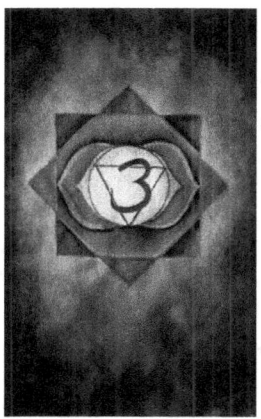

It is located between the eyebrows in the center of the forehead. This is the center of intuition, wisdom & awareness. Ajna is associated with the mind.

The brow or third eye chakra deals with perceiving and psychic power. It is the sixth chakra associated with the color indigo which represents intuition.

Functions of the Ajna Chakra/Third Eye Chakra

Physical

The third eye chakra governs the face, the pineal and pituitary gland, eyes, nose, ears and the skeletal system. It improves memory, develops ability to distinguish between reality and imagination. A person with a strong ajna chakra can rely on his intuition, perception and interpretation. It increase focus, clarity, harmony and well-being.

If the third eye chakra is blocked it might cause headaches/migraines, sinus, brain tumors, strokes, blindness, deafness, learning disabilities, spinal dysfunctions, depression, fear of truth, confusion, and even poor eye sightedness. It might even result in high blood pressure, low immune system, acute sinusitis and anxiousness.

Emotions

When well balanced you see things clearly, not only physically, but also morally. It is related to your ability, to perceive and shape your own opinions about what you see and how you feel.

When blocked you feel frustrated, irritated, can't make proper decision, misunderstandings, nightmares, headaches, insensitivity, lack of concentration, bad memory, lack of imagination, difficulty visualizing and emotional problems surround you.

Addictions

Living in imaginary world, exaggeration, perceptual defense.

Spiritual

This chakra mainly focuses on **Insight**, if balanced; you see and perceive things clearly. "**Clarity**" is the key to clear any blockages related to Ajna chakra. Breakthrough *"Illusion",* see things/ situation clearly before you react or assume something. Learn to see from all the angles.

Meditation, coloring and drawing, learning any sort of art, working with memory, watching fishes swim and feeding them or nature walks help to clear blocks related to ajna chakra.

☐ Sahasrara Chakra/Crown Chakra

Sahasrara is described as a thousand-petaled lotus, located at the top/crown of the head. This relates to pure consciousness & one's personal & spiritual connection to the universe. Typically associates with pineal, pituitary gland & the spiritual world.

The crown chakra or Sahasrara is the last of the seven main chakras and is represented by the color violet. It is mainly related to spirituality, it is the connection to the divine energy. It is also called as lotus with one thousand petals.

Functions of the Sahasrara Chakra/Crown Chakra

Physical

The crown chakra governs many organs and glands of the body such as the brain, the nervous system and the pituitary gland. Balanced crown chakra connects us to the divine power easily. It enables us to receive clear intuition/guidance, wisdom, mastery, broad understanding and awareness, ability to perceive, analyze and assimilate information from the higher source.

An imbalanced crown chakra may cause problems such as migraines, coma, stroke, brain tumors, amnesia and cognitive delusions. Also increases stress, learning difficulties, anxiety, hysteria and depression.

Emotions

When well balanced we feel positivity, trust, happiness, truth, peace and feeling of oneness. Unconditional love, compassion, wisdom are essential part of this chakra.

An imbalanced crown chakra revolves around issues like lack of reality, loss of purpose or meaning in one's life, ego problems, lack of knowledge, lack of acceptance and concern for oneself and others, being judgmental and rude in nature, rigid belief systems, materialism, greed.

Addictions

Religion, spiritual practices, Ego.

Spiritual

It connects to your higher self and opens up love and compassion towards all. This chakra mainly focuses on cosmic energy.

"**Divine wisdom, detachment along with compassion towards all**" is the key to clear any blockages related to Sahasrara chakra. Divine wisdom comes in the purest form without any ego and pride. It teaches us to see all as one and unique at the same time. Drop your "**ego**" or any "**worldly attachments**". Knowledge flows through you so be thankful for selecting you.

Learn to be compassionate and detached at the same time. Share knowledge, never stop learning, respect all irrespective of age, caste and creed.

Chakras	Physical level	Emotional level	spiritual level		
	Deals with	Related Organs	Deals with	Blocked by	

Sahasrara Chakra	Intuition	Pineal gland / brain	Divine Wisdom	Ego / Attachment	Cosmic energy
Ajna Chakra	Memory	Eye and head	Clarity	Illusion	Insight
Vishuddha Chakra	Communication	Thymus and Thyroid	Self-expression	Lies	Truth
Anahata Chakra	Relationship	Heart	Understanding	Grief	Love

Manipura Chakra	Vitality	Stomach	Strength	Disgrace	Will power
Swadhisthana Chakra	Feelings	Reproductive organs	Passion	Guilt	Pleasure
Muladhara Chakra	Finance/material - wellbeing	Kidneys, bladder, spine	Trust	Fear	Survival

Chapter 18: Reiki Practice And Growth Of Intuitive Abilities

By Deborah Lloyd

One memory I have of my Reiki training was my Master's beautiful warning: "Get ready. If you use Reiki frequently, your life will change very quickly. It can be an awesome ride." One common area where many of us Reiki practitioners have grown is the opening of the third eye – and that is an awesome ride.

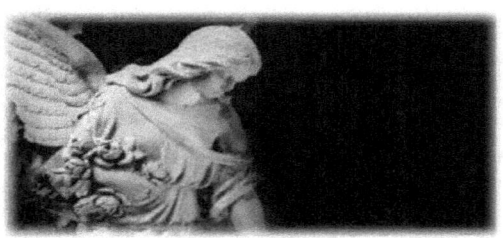

During a session within several months of completing my Master training, and the opening of our healing center, I saw, in my mind's eye, a healing angel walk into the room and do Reiki with me. She worked on the client's legs and feet, when my hands were around the client's head. When I moved to the lower portion of the body, the angel worked on the upper. I wondered if it was real, or simply my imagination.

My question was answered when the client shared her experience. She said the session was wonderful, and she thought a second practitioner had joined us. She reported she opened her eyes several times as she felt two pairs of hands on her body; she described exactly the various positions of both the angel and me. I asked if she believed in angels, and she did; so, I shared my vision with her. She was astounded!

And, so was I. At that time, I had not considered the possibility that I would be able to "see" any spiritual being, or ever be able to develop that capacity. I thought people who had that talent were few, specifically chosen by the Universe to bring healing messages to others in this unique way. What I did not realize is that every person has intuitive abilities, and each of us can grow in that capacity. The more you learn and practice – and believe in the possibility – the greater your intuition can grow.

Reiki can put you on the fast track of intuitive development. Set your intention and place your hands on the third eye chakra, daily. Invite Spirit Guides to work with you, while you are giving Reiki to others, or to yourself. Read the stories of the famous psychics and mediums. You'll soon learn that each one doubted their abilities, in their early days. They did not think they were special enough, or good enough, or a multitude of other "not enough's." These intuitives are simply normal people, who are open to accepting this gift. Use Reiki to help yourself reach your full potential in intuitive abilities.

Increasing the energy flow of any chakra affects the chakras on either side of it, bringing more energetic balance to the body. It is no coincidence that the third eye chakra borders the crown chakra. As the third eye opens, the spiritual connection is strengthened. As the connection to Spirit grows, the third eye chakra opens even more – and a lovely cycle has begun, and can continue for a lifetime, if intention and positive energy continues. Practice this frequently – and enjoy the awesome ride.

10 Tips to Find Time for Daily Practice

Finding the time for daily self-Reiki can be challenging, especially for new practitioners, or busy people who have a lot going on in their lives.

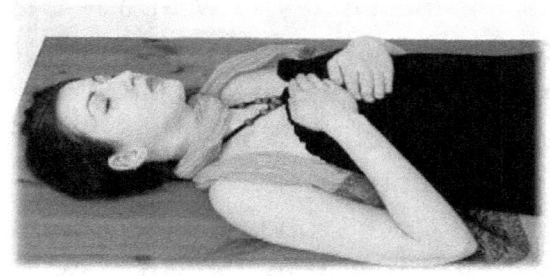

Here are some tips to help you get past that initial stage when new tasks and new things to do seem to just come up out of nowhere, leaving you no time for yourself. After you keep practicing for several days, you'll find that it gets easier to find the time, and after a few weeks, it even becomes easier to keep Reiki-ing :) than not to.

Tip 1. Practice before going to bed. If you're very tired, just go to bed, place a hand on your third eye chakra, and one on your heart, and send Reiki. It's OK to fall asleep.

Tip 2. Wake up earlier. Yes, it's challenging, but definitely worth it. Waking up 10-15 minutes earlier and doing 1 minute of Reiki in each hand positions will have a great impact in the long term.

Tip 3. Use the "idle" time, e.g. on the train, waiting in line at the bank...

Tip 4. Send Reiki to yourself or your situation with the intent that you manage to find more time for practicing.

Tip 5. Ask your guides, or your subconscious mind, to help you solve the time problem. Just stay open to any solution - and you'll be surprised to see how quickly it works :).

Tip 6. Set an appointment with yourself, every day, and make it highest priority. Treat it like a flight you absolutely have to be on.

Tip 7. Send Reiki to your Solar Plexus Chakra - this is the chakra of personal power, which governs the power of your will among others. A strong will will help you find solutions and prioritize things that are important for you, personally.

Tip 8. Find a "Reiki buddy" that you practice together with - it will increase the accountability and you'll both have a better chance sticking to the schedule.

Tip 9. *Place a time-related affirmation in your Reiki box, such as* I always have enough time to do everything I desire, for my highest good.

Tip 10. Reduce time spent on other activities, such as TV, internet browsing, Facebook, email.

Conclusion

The amount of exercises that I have included has been limited to beginner exercises. Don't try to move forward too quickly. Once you have learned these exercises, you can go on to learn even more. The most important from my point of view is going to be your practice at meditation as this is what gives you that wonderful sense of peace and of knowing yourself. It also helps you to gain self-confidence and to feel at peace with those around you, which is probably the most important thing that you can glean from yoga.

If you find that you cannot concentrate sufficiently to meditate correctly, then it may be an idea to try concentrating on a mantra such as the word Ohm. This helps to shut out thoughts that are stopping you from meditating. To say the word Ohm correctly, you need to have your lips slightly apart and chant it as you meditate and it should cause a tingle on your lips. If it does not, try it again with the mouth a little more open until it does. This is a good practice for people with ultra-busy minds that are hard to shut down by other means. It may also be what you need in order to achieve meditation. If you want something to help you to get the pitch to your liking, you can buy a Tibetan singing bowl and before your meditation, use this to sing out the note for you. There are various models available on the Internet and you don't need to spend a lot either.

Another alternative for those who don't like counting when they are meditating is to invest in meditation beads and instead of concentrating on counting, you can pass the beads through your fingers until you reach the end of the beads, at which time, your meditation session is over.

This book was written for absolute beginners, but I hope that I have enthused you a little, or at least enough to give meditation and yoga a try. It isn't hard. It doesn't demand more of you than you are able to give, but what it gives back is much more than any exercise program ever will. It gives you back a lifestyle that is caring and that means that you will find peace as a result of the work that you do. I have known many people who have taken up yoga and who have struggled with the meditation part of it all. If you do find this hard, try relaxation exercises where you lie down and concentrate on different parts of the body that you tense and then relax. This usually covers from your toes right up to the top of your head. You simply close your eyes, feel that part of the body that you want to concentrate on, flex it and then relax it, before moving on to the next part of your body. What this does is give you something alternative to think about instead of simply thinking about your breathing. However, if you do this, remember that comfort is important and that you should think of nothing else at all.

It is hoped that you have learned something and that you are able to sit down and do these exercises and feel good about them. I love waking in the morning and doing the sun salutation because I feel it brings me closer to my spiritual side. I do this on a beach or in an outdoor area because it inspires me. You can too and when you do, you will find that your whole outlook on life will change for the better and that you will find that peace that it is that you crave. The journey in yoga is a continual one where you are always growing and always learning. As I said at the beginning, you don't do yoga, you live it. That's when it hits you that your life has changed beyond recognition, but in a very positive way.

www.ingramcontent.com/pod-product-compliance
Lightning Source LLC
Chambersburg PA
CBHW072004070526
44583CB00015B/1328